I AM ROCK STEADY

Fighting Back Against Parkinson's Disease

Inspirational stories about the courageous boxers of
Rock Steady Boxing as told to Julie Young

First published by Dog Ear Publishing
4011 Vincennes Rd
Indianapolis, IN 46268
www.dogearpublishing.net

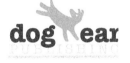

ISBN: 978-1-4575-4890-1

This book is printed on acid-free paper.

Printed in the United States of America

CONTENTS

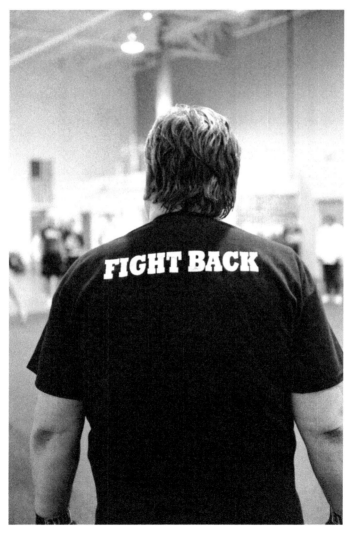

Preface

"It ain't about how hard you hit; it's about how hard you can get hit
and keep moving forward…
that's how winning is done."
—Rocky Balboa

As a writer and author, I am asked to collaborate on any number of book-related projects throughout the year. Very few of them pan out. There are several reasons why this occurs. In most cases, I am simply not the best writer for the job. I may lack the expertise necessary to complete the research to pen an entire volume on a specific subject. The production schedule may be time-sensitive and not something I can add to my calendar. There may be a conflict of interest or other compelling reason for me not to get involved with a particular project, but every once in a while, I am presented with an idea so intriguing, I simply have to be a part of it.

That was the case in February 2015 when Joyce Johnson, Executive Director of Rock Steady Boxing, Inc., contacted me to ask if I would be interested in writing a book about an exercise program designed to help folks fight back against Parkinson's disease. She said she hoped to create a book full of inspirational stories that would not only promote interest in the Rock Steady Boxing program itself but also showcase the amazing and courageous men and women who were using the program as a way to delay, reduce, and even reverse the symptoms of their condition.

At first, I wasn't sure what to think. Nearly everything I knew about boxing came straight out of the *Rocky* franchise, and my working knowledge of Parkinson's was limited to a rudimentary definition and a handful of famous names associated with the affliction. I was pretty sure that the idea of a boxing program created to help people with Parkinson's was a contradiction in terms. After all, wasn't boxing the reason Muhammad Ali developed Parkinson's in the first place?

Amused that an organization would align itself with a sport so closely (and negatively) connected to a condition it was trying to fight, I agreed to drive out to the Rock Steady Boxing headquarters in Indianapolis to see the program in action. I assumed it would be a kind of watered-down chair aerobics class that resembled boxing in name only, but I was wrong. Dead wrong. When I walked into the sunny yellow Rock Steady Boxing gym in Indianapolis for the first time, I could not believe my eyes. It was a real boxing gym just like in the movies, complete with a full-size ring, speed bags, heavy bags, gloves, and more.

Led Zeppelin's "Kashmir" blasted over the sound system as a small, muscular woman in a bandana barked orders to her boxers, sounding like a cross between a drill sergeant and an angry parent. She scared me to death, but none of her fighters ran screaming for the doors. As a matter of fact, they seemed to respond to her particular brand of tough talk! *What in the world is going on here?* I wondered.

As I watched the class in progress, I was amazed by the diversity of the people in the room. There was an even mix of men and women among the attendees, and a wide range of ages. Only one fit my chair-aerobic stereotype, but even she packed some pretty solid punches against her cornerman's mitts. During the tour, the Executive Director Joyce pointed out a healthy-looking gentleman working on the heavy bag and told me how much he had improved since he had started the program.

"He has Parkinson's?" I asked incredulously. "I thought he was a coach!"

The incredible thing about the Rock Steady Boxing program is not only its effectiveness in battling the symptoms of Parkinson's disease but also the men and women who are part of it. When they are training in the gym, they are no longer Parkinson's patients. They are boxers fighting for their lives, and make no mistake about it, they are giving it everything they've got. When I left the gym that day, I was full of excitement about the journey ahead and could not wait to get started.

The men and women you will meet in this book are some of the most courageous and inspiring people it's been my pleasure to know. They come from a variety of locations around the world and have very different backgrounds and experiences, yet they are forever bonded by a condition they never bargained for and by a will to survive. These boxers pull no punches in telling their stories, and I invite you now to step into the ring with me to meet some of the fighters of Rock Steady Boxing … a group sure to knock you out!

—Julie Young, 2016

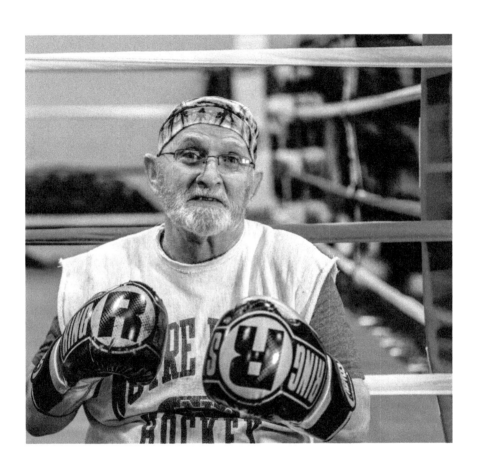

INTRODUCTION

"Boxing is easy. Life is much harder."
—Floyd Mayweather Jr.

Parkinson's disease is a progressive disorder of the nervous system that affects one's ability to move. The condition occurs when the neurons in the substantia nigra portion of the brain die off, rendering it unable to produce and deliver dopamine to the rest of the organ. Although it is unclear what causes the death of these neurons, several factors are believed to play a part, including one's genes, environment, mental triggers, and the presence of Lewy bodies—specific material within one's brain cells that are tiny markers for the condition.

Parkinson's affects 7–10 million people worldwide and typically begins when one is middle-aged or older, although it can occur in someone much younger. Michael J. Fox, for example, was diagnosed at the age of 29. Parkinson's develops gradually and often begins with slight, nearly imperceptible signs such as a small tremor in one hand or leg, or along one side of the body. Other early symptoms include stiffness in the limbs, slowed movement, and lack of facial expression. Although the individual indicators may vary and no two cases are exactly alike, patients may experience painful muscle spasms, may struggle with a lack of coordination, and may find themselves unable to perform basic tasks. They are prone to depression and falls and, in the later stages, may experience delusions and have difficulty swallowing food.

Indiana University neurologist Dr. Joanne Wojcieszek says by the time a patient notices the initial symptoms of Parkinson's and addresses his or her concerns with a doctor, 80 percent of the dopamine-producing neurons are dead; after that, progression of symptoms is a race against the clock. Medications such as carbidopa-levodopa, Duodopa, MAO-B inhibitors, and more can help stimulate the dopamine effect in the body, but doctors also recommend exercise as well as mental stimulation to keep the body strong and the mind alert. Despite these weapons to keep the condition and its symptoms at bay, there is no known cure for Parkinson's, and once diagnosed, patients are told they have only about 10 productive years left.

One of the highest-profile Parkinson's cases, and the one most people are familiar with aside from Michael J. Fox is that of Muhammad Ali, the former heavyweight champion of the world. Ali was diagnosed with Parkinson's in 1984 at the age of 42, but because he exhibited signs of the disease not long after retiring from the professional ring in 1981, it was widely believed that his boxing career somehow caused the condition to occur. Although it is possible that one too many blows to the head may have contributed to Ali's illness, Dr. Abraham Lieberman, Ali's personal physician, said in 2014 that it is impossible to know for sure what ultimately led to the legendary fighter's affliction. "It's very difficult to factor in what sort of role did boxing play," he said.

It is true that there is a higher risk for Parkinson's disease among boxers, but there is also a higher risk of Parkinson's in any sport or activity that can result in repeated head trauma, including football, hockey, and martial arts. Nonetheless, the misconception persists that boxing and Parkinson's are intrinsically related—a misconception that the folks at Rock Steady Boxing have fought hard to overcome.

Joyce Johnson, Executive Director of Rock Steady Boxing, Inc., understands the initial reservations that people may have about the program when they first hear about it. When one of the most well-known Parkinson's patients happens to be one of the most beloved and iconic fighters of all time, it's no surprise that boxing is the sport that comes to mind when someone hears the term "Parkinson's disease."

"Rock Steady Boxing was founded in 2006 by a former Marion County Prosecutor and is a *noncontact* program that uses traditional boxing techniques to give people hope while improving their quality of life," Johnson says. "Boxers condition for optimal agility, speed, and overall strength in order to defeat their opponent. At Rock Steady Boxing, our boxers do the same thing, but in this case, the opponent is Parkinson's disease."

Various studies in the 1980s and 1990s supported the idea that exercise that emphasizes gross motor movement, balance, core strength, rhythm, and hand-eye coordination has a favorable impact on range of motion, flexibility, posture, gait, and everyday activities. More recent studies, most notably one at the Cleveland Clinic, focus on the concept of intense "forced" exercise and suggest that certain types of exercise are neuro-protective, meaning they may actually slow disease progression.

At Rock Steady Boxing, stretches are used to help with muscle stiffness. Footwork promotes balance. Punching serves to steady the tremors. Yelling strengthens the vocal chords, and hitting focus mitts encourages better coordination. Boxers and clinicians alike say that they can see a vast improvement in motor skills, speech, and sensory function, and with more than 200 affiliate locations (and growing) throughout the world, Rock Steady Boxing is sure to be a contender in the fight against Parkinson's for years to come.

"Discovery of a cure may be years away, but at Rock Steady Boxing, our boxers can do something to fight back," said Johnson.

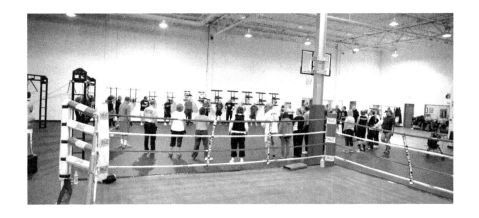

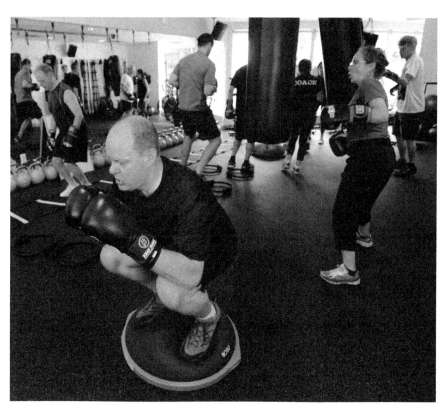

Rock Steady Boxing Vancouver, B.C.

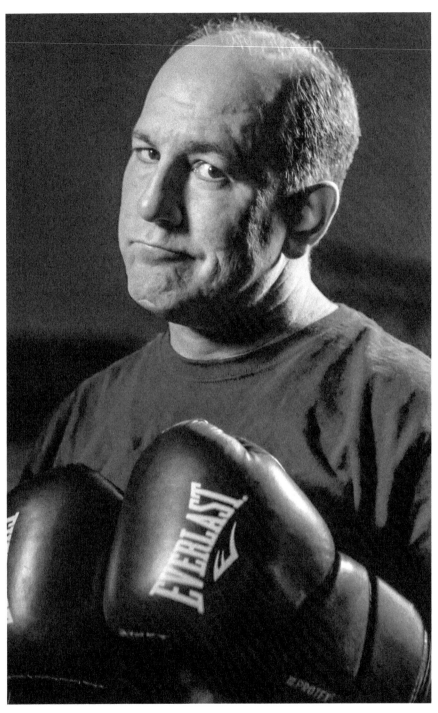

Scott Newman, Founder
Rock Steady Boxing

ROUND 1

A Shaky Future

"A champion is someone who gets up when he can't."
—Jack Dempsey

Scott Newman always had a flair for the dramatic. A native of Chicago's suburbs, he was a natural showman who regaled his friends in the school yard with his special brand of playground shtick. At the age of 11, he launched his own magic business with a friend and began appearing at backyard birthday parties. During his high school graduation speech, he offered up a wild and crazy impression of *Saturday Night Live* funnyman Steve Martin, but it was in the courtroom where Scott parlayed his penchant for performance into his public crusade for truth and justice. It was also the place where he unwittingly began his personal battle with Parkinson's disease.

Scott was not merely amusing. He was also an academic. After he completed his undergraduate work at Princeton and received his law degree from Michigan, most of his family and friends assumed the wunderkind would waltz off to Wall Street, where he could earn millions a year in the private sector. They were surprised when Scott eschewed the idea of a cushy life in corporate law and opted instead for a life in public service.

A few, such as his father, who was also an attorney, went so far as to express doubts about Scott's career choice. "He said I wouldn't last a year when I found out how unglamorous it was," Scott recalled in a 2003 interview.

But Scott would not be dissuaded. He applied for prosecutor positions in Florida as well as in several states in the Midwest. He wanted to make a name for himself in a medium-sized city, and when Marion County Prosecutor Stephen Goldsmith received Scott's resume, he arranged to interview the fellow Michigan alum who had gotten better grades than he had. After meeting Scott and vetting his qualifications, Goldsmith offered Scott a job. Scott accepted and relocated to Indianapolis, Indiana.

In Indianapolis, Scott hit the ground running and learned on the job, handling a number of high-profile cases. "It blew my mind that right out of law school, without passing 'Go,' I got to handle cases that were on the front page of the newspaper, up against some of the best lawyers in the city," he said.

In 1988, the young prosecutor became an assistant US attorney under Deborah Daniels. It was a six-year stint that introduced Scott to his mentor Larry Mackey and enabled him to hone his preparation skills and emotionally connect with a jury during a case. It also led to his decision to run for the position of Marion County prosecutor on the GOP ticket in 1994.

As with his decision to enter public service, not everyone thought this a wise move, and few thought he stood a chance against the Democratic incumbent Jeff Modisett.

One of the naysayers was Stephen Goldsmith, the former prosecutor who had given Scott his first job. "When he came to me, I thought, 'This will not work.' He had the barnacles of being associated with me. He had no rational political base. And he was an out-of-towner. That campaign was just short of hopeless," Goldsmith said in 2003.

Hopeless or not, Scott persevered, and it wasn't long before he found voters who responded to his get-tough-on-crime message. His popularity grew, and although he was down 2-1 to his opponent in pre-election polls, he won the race by 6,000 votes. Four years later, he would be reelected in a landslide.

Throughout his legal career, Scott never hesitated to employ attention-grabbing theatrics and his own unique brand of humor to get his point across. During the closing arguments of a complicated and controversial corruption case, he compared summarizing the wealth of evidence to cleaning up the Exxon Valdez oil spill with a simple mop. After listening to a defense attorney plead for the life of a convicted cop-killer during sentencing, he wafted tissues in the air and directed the jury to cry over the officer who had lost his life. In one memorable case, which involved the death of another policeman, Scott illustrated the weight of losing a public servant by dropping a bowling ball on the courtroom floor. "It was really effective in getting the message across to the jury," recalled Marion County Superior Court Judge Patricia Gifford.

The event that made the most impact—on Scott, anyway—occurred in April of 1999. He was summing up his closing argument against a defendant who had killed a six-year-old in a drug deal, and when he slapped a $20 bill in front of the man as if to say that was the only value the man placed on human life, Scott felt his whole left side tremble. Assuming it was a physical reaction to the intensity of the moment, he thought, *Hey, that's pretty cool.*

It was anything but cool, though; over the next two years, his symptoms continued and worsened. At times, his left hand shook involuntarily. His arm was stiff. His typing speed slowed, and his wife began to notice similar issues in his leg. When she pointed it out to him, Scott tried to dismiss her concern. "I've always had that," he told her.

Despite his brave words, Scott knew something was wrong, and deep down, he knew what it had to be. He'd seen the same symptoms in others, including former US Attorney General Janet Reno, so when he was officially diagnosed with young-onset Parkinson's disease in October 2001 at the age of 40, he wasn't too surprised. He also wasn't fazed by what many would consider to be a devastating diagnosis, though he would later attribute his blasé attitude to a lack of knowledge about his condition. "I thought it was an irritating tremor, something you could live with indefinitely. But the more I've learned, the scarier it's gotten," he said.

Scott consulted with Indiana University Neurologist and Movement Disorder Specialist Dr. Joanne Wojcieszek, who put him on a dopamine agonist for quick relief of his symptoms, and he began working out with Denise Austin's television show each morning. Because of the public nature of his job, Scott understandably chose to keep his condition private. He shared the news with those it was absolutely necessary to tell and relied on a number of Parkinson's tricks to get him through various events. He kept his hand inside his jacket pocket during appearances and signed documents in his office rather than risk shaky signing ceremonies, but as his symptoms progressed, he knew his secret would not stay hidden forever.

Rumors were already starting to spread. Coworkers and members of the press spotted his hand shaking at a fundraising event and speculated that he had Parkinson's, but Scott knew if he wanted the news of his condition to come out on his own terms, he needed to address the issue. He'd already made the decision not to seek a third term, and he wanted to let his prospective employers know about his situation prior to hiring him. He also wanted to make sure the public knew that his physical condition did not have a bearing on his decision to not seek reelection. He prosecuted one final high-profile case just as the news of his condition broke on September 24, 2002.

The public reaction to Scott's condition was nothing short of overwhelming, as cards, e-mails, and shout-outs poured in from all over. He said it was a relief to have the news out in the open at last. "What I was hiding was the fact that I was vulnerable … I wasn't superhuman if, indeed, anyone thought I was," he said.

Although Scott tried to handle his diagnosis with his typical pragmatism and self-deprecating sense of humor, he admits there were plenty of low moments as well. It was frustrating when his medications left him feeling fatigued, when he had to start relying on voice-activated software in order to type, and when he didn't feel as if he were getting enough from his daily workouts. After leaving office, Scott admitted, he fell into a period of inactivity and apathy regarding his disease. "I was ready to throw in the towel," he said. "Parkinson's disease … was pummeling me into a shadow of my former self. I had hit the canvas. I took to my bed and my cringing self-pity, and I felt sure that my Creator was calling the count over my increasingly lifeless body."

It looked like a technical knockout for sure, but out of nowhere, Vincent "Vince" Perez stepped in and changed Scott's life forever. Vince was a cop turned lawyer and former Golden Gloves champion who was loathe to see his friend withdrawing from life so completely. He came in out of nowhere and told Scott that he was going to teach Scott how to box, in hopes that it would help. "He said, 'I am your cornerman. I am your trainer. Now, get up!'"

Vince and Scott began their intense one-on-one workouts in which Vince shamed, trained, punished, and insulted Scott into fighting for his life. At first, Scott said, he was very uncoordinated, partially because of the Parkinson's and partially because of the unfamiliarity of the workout. Vince worked him without mercy for five and six days a week, and gradually, Scott began to see an improvement in his symptoms. "An amazing thing was happening. I was getting better: physically stronger, quicker, more flexible, more alert, more confident. … All of this without adding a single microgram of the side-effect-ridden medication for Parkinson's."

Vince also noticed a change in Scott, in terms of both his physical stamina and his mental attitude. Dr. Wojcieszek noted improvement as well and encouraged Scott to keep doing whatever he was doing, knowing that vigorous and regular exercise could have a positive impact on his symptoms, including his stiffness and slowness, and on his agility and overall sense of well-being.

As Vince's boxing workouts continued to improve

Scott's quality of life, the pair talked about sharing their technique with other Parkinson's patients in hopes it could help them as well. In 2006, they opened a small borrowed gym on the east side of Indianapolis that was funded by private donations and open free of charge to anyone who could climb inside the ring. At dinner one evening, Scott held out his arms straight in front of him. He was tremor-free and said, "Look, I'm rock steady!" So they chose the name Rock Steady Boxing for this new venture.

The goal of the Rock Steady Boxing program was to provide a place where those affected by Parkinson's disease could feel comfortable and gain confidence in their abilities. By being part of this program, people with Parkinson's can go out and live day-to-day life in the real world.

The Rock Steady Boxing program provides a combination of endurance, strength, power, speed, agility, flexibility, durability, and hand-eye coordination exercises with that same blend of respect and tough talk that Vince initially gave Scott. Although the trainers are not always "nice," they are committed to each trainee and offer plenty of high hopes, constant challenge, and loads of support. "Here no one is ashamed of his or her symptoms, and all share a commitment to fighting their way off the ropes and finishing strong in life, as in each round of a boxing match," Scott said.

Within the first two years of Rock Steady Boxing's existence, there were enough trainees for Scott and Vince to hire more coaches to help out with the dozens of prospects finding their way to the gym. The job description was simple: Scott wanted a female professional boxer with a winning record who was great with people of all ages and had a heart for those with disabilities. He found all that in former second-ranked, world-champion boxer Kristina "Kristy" Rose Follmar.

Kristy Rose Follmar

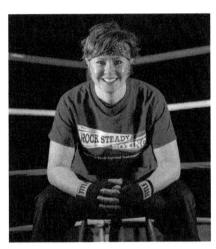

Kristy Rose Follmar

Kristy was born in Cedar Lake, Indiana, into a typical close-knit, happy, loving family that included her parents, one sibling, and numerous aunts, uncles, and cousins. At the age of 13, however, she endured a blow that no young person should have to face so early in life: the tragic and untimely death of her father, Donald.

"Out of nowhere, my father committed suicide," she told a newspaper reporter in 2004. "When my mom broke it to me, I just remember getting so completely ... mad that I wanted to hit something. My mom happened to be standing right in front of me. I don't even remember doing it, but I guess I whacked her."

To help her daughter cope with her feelings of loss, anger, and frustration, Kristy's mother bought her a heavy bag and gloves and encouraged Kristy to go for it. Kristy found that hitting the bag was more therapeutic than keeping her emotions bottled up inside or taking them out on those around her, but she didn't get serious about the sport until she was a sophomore at Ball State University and started working out at the Muncie Police Athletic League (PAL) Club.

Kristy's first boxing competition was a Toughman Contest, which is an event that gives novice fighters the chance to prove themselves in the ring. The Toughman Contest uses standard boxing rules but has shorter rounds and contains more safety gear and precautions than a traditional match. Created by promoter Art Dore in 1979, it is an iconic event in the world of boxing and has helped spark the careers of future Rocky costars Mr. T (Rocky III) and Tommy Morrison (Rocky V).

Kristy's raw talent eventually caught the eye of trainers Mark Lemerick and Rodney Cummings, who took her under their wing. Under their guidance, she went 7-1 as an amateur before making her professional debut on February 26, 2002, at Pepsi Coliseum in Indianapolis. Her opponent was Annie Briant of Martinsville, who was also making her debut that evening. Kristy KO'd Briant in the first round, which not only caused the judges to sit up and take notice but also established her throughout the boxing community as a star on the rise.

By the time she retired in 2005, Kristy was a college graduate who boasted a professional boxing record of 15-1, with nine knockouts to her credit. She not only was an Indiana Golden Gloves Women's Champ but also went on to become the first-ever Women's Indiana State Champion, NABC Featherweight, and Super Featherweight World Champion. Not long after her last official fight in March 2005 against Kim Colbert, however, Kristy learned that she was expecting a baby. She hung up the gloves and put boxing on the back burner to plunge headfirst into motherhood. She gave birth to a daughter, Kay O'Connor, affectionately nicknamed Baby KO.

When Kristy learned that Scott was looking for an executive director for his boxing facility in Indianapolis, the 26-year-old was not sure she was the right person for the job. Although she had a degree in telecommunications/marketing and sociology, the credentials to be a top-notch trainer, and a boxing record many fighters would die for, she thought it might be depressing to be around people with Parkinson's disease all day, every day. She worried that she might come home mentally and physically drained, with nothing left to give her daughter, but after meeting several of the Rock Steady clients, she realized nothing could be further from the truth. If anything, the men and women she encountered each day helped to keep her spirits high with their tenacity, strength, and can-do attitude. "I mean, these people are just fighters," she said in an April 2008 newspaper interview.

Just when everything was going well, tragedy once again struck Kristy's family. On September 17, 2008, her 23-year-old brother, Thomas, ended his life. Just as she had when she was a teenager, Kristy turned to boxing in order to deal with her grief. She made the decision to come out of retirement and face South Bend native Eva Jones-Young for the Women's WBF World Light Welterweight Championship on March 3, 2009.

"When my brother died, I had a really hard time for the first couple months snapping back into reality and finding motivation to work," Kristy said. "Then this fight came up, and even though I had made the decision to hang it up and focus on my family, I felt like it would give me something else to focus on."

Kristy won the bout in a decisive victory and returned to the ring a month later to take on Mary McGee of Gary for the WBO World Title at the Civic Center in Hammond. Though she would lose the match in a split decision, many remembered the event as one of the best women's professional boxing matchups in the sport's history. She retired for a second time in 2010 with a 16-2 record.

Kristy has been with Rock Steady as program director and head coach for 10 years, and she says it is gratifying to see so many people triumph as a result of the program. Being around the fighters at Rock Steady has shown her that when something bad happens in life, you can still smile, be happy, and fight. "The commitment and dedication displayed by the people in our program is inspirational," she said. "They've become like family to me."

As word of the program spread and demand for classes increased, Rock Steady Boxing created a unique training program to meet the fitness levels at all stages of Parkinson's disease, from the newly diagnosed to those who have been living with their condition for decades or more. Participants discovered that boxing training not only offered an appropriately challenging workout but was also fun! Rock Steady boxers found a place where, inside and outside of the ring, they could form friendships with others who truly understood what it was like to live with Parkinson's disease.

"Here at Rock Steady Boxing, every day is different. There's jump rope, speed bags, you name it," Kristy said. "We offer a great variety in our workouts. The body movements in our workouts help out Parkinson's people who have mobility issues. It gets emotional when you see the improvements. And the pride in their eyes. It's a great thing to see."

As for the former prosecutor who started it all, although he knows Parkinson's is a battle he may eventually lose, the future is not as shaky as it once was, and he's not about to go down without a fight. "Parkinson's is a clinical thing you can deal with. And I've taken it on pretty successfully. It can be managed. If your head is in the wrong place, then it can't be managed. How you deal with the inevitable is the mark of quality in a man or woman. It's not bravery; it's necessity," Scott said. "Starting a boxing gym specifically for people with Parkinson's disease to fight back is one of the most rewarding things I have done with my career."

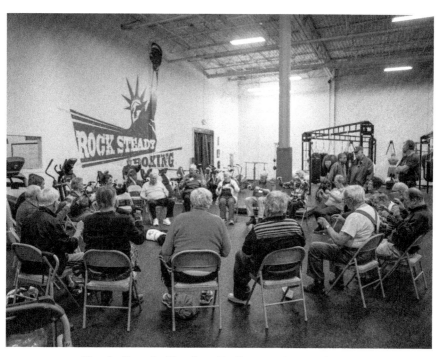

Rock Steady Boxing Indianapolis, Indiana

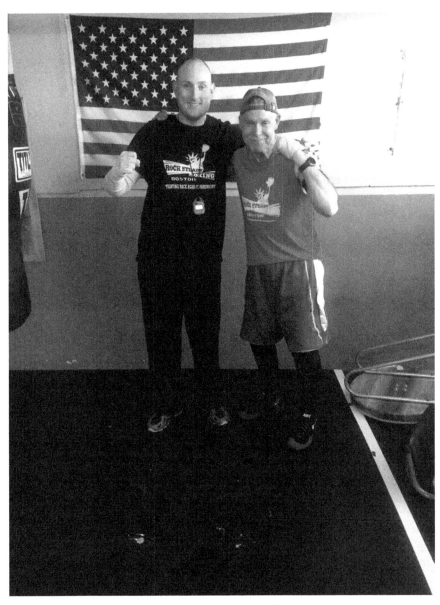

Greg Geheb and Coach Al Latulippe
Rock Steady Boxing Boston

ROUND 2

It's Now or Never

"If you train hard and responsibly your confidence surges to the maximum."
—Floyd Patterson

Long before he discovered Rock Steady Boxing, Greg Geheb of Nashua, New Hampshire, was accustomed to slugging it out day after day. As a software engineer who worked on Lotus 1-2-3/M and Lotus Notes for IBM, he labored in a highly competitive and pressure-filled environment where products must be pushed, employees often competed for recognition, and two bad evaluations in a row could be your last.

"It was a sedentary job, but an intense one, and when I began falling behind in 2008, I knew I was down for the count," he said. "It was only a matter of time before my supervisor knew it as well."

The diminished productivity was the latest in a long line of issues that had plagued Greg over the past decade and left him feeling like a shell of his former self. Ever since he had begun working from home in the mid-'00s, he hadn't been as active as he once had, and it was no secret that the lower activity levels had taken a toll on his general health. At 260 pounds, he was considered obese, could no longer walk as fast he used to, and had taken to sleeping on the sofa instead of in his bed at night. His wife, Kathy, joked that he was getting lazy with age, but Greg sensed that wasn't the problem. He didn't enjoy sleeping on the sofa, but he couldn't get comfortable anywhere else. The blankets felt unbearably heavy, and it was next to impossible for him to roll over. Greg also shuffled when he puttered about the house and had a slight tremor in his hand that was noticeable when he Skyped with his grandsons.

Greg took his concerns to his primary care physician, an experienced doctor who recognized the signs and promptly sent him to a neurologist for evaluation. After a few consultations and an MRI, the specialist gave it to him straight: Greg had young-onset Parkinson's disease. "I was officially diagnosed on February 9, 2009," he said. "Come to find out, all of the problems I was experiencing were classic symptoms of the condition. I was the poster child for Parkinson's, but I didn't know it at the time."

In truth, Greg didn't know much about Parkinson's disease at all. Although the doctor told him it was not fatal and that with a proper treatment plan, including medication and exercise, he would be able to enjoy a full and productive life, it was obvious he could no longer keep up with the demands of his fast-paced career. He tried to continue working for a period of time after his diagnosis, but his hand cramped as he tried to move the computer mouse, his cognitive skills began to suffer, and he continued to fall behind his colleagues. In September of 2009, Greg reluctantly left his position at IBM and was placed on long-term disability. It was a difficult decision that left him feeling useless and more than a little depressed. The job he had thought he would have until retirement was gone, and in its place was a full-time gig in disease management. It wasn't exactly a fair trade-off.

Nevertheless, Greg took on his new role and began researching his condition. Although his medical team had stressed the importance of exercise to keep his symptoms in check, they had never specified what type of exercise would be most beneficial. Greg couldn't find anything on the Internet either, but he knew he had to do something. He ultimately joined the local YMCA, where he worked out on the weight machines and elliptical, rode the recumbent bike, and walked around the track, but he didn't see a substantial improvement. He lost weight. He regained some of his stamina, but he didn't get the big boost he was hoping for. After three years of this routine, Greg was discouraged and depressed. "I thought, *Here I am, 60 years old. I have a wife and two grown children to live for. I have four grandchildren, and I want to dance at their weddings.* I wasn't sleeping well. I was tired all the time, and I knew my symptoms were only getting worse."

In November 2012, Greg traveled to Indianapolis, Indiana, to visit his daughter Abby and her family for the Thanksgiving holiday. Always one to promote fitness and exercise, Abby couldn't wait to tell her father about a program she'd discovered that was designed for people with Parkinson's disease—Rock Steady Boxing. It was based locally and was getting rave reviews. Abby had even talked to one colleague of her husband, Ted, at the University of Indianapolis about it. Dr. Stephanie Combs-Miller, a physical therapy professor, had begun researching the positive effects of the Rock Steady Boxing program on Parkinson's patients. Abby was convinced it would work for her father and asked him to give it a shot. Although Greg had never boxed a round in his life and was nervous about the prospect of going toe-to-toe with anyone, he agreed to give it a try. He said he would have done anything at that point if he thought it would help him get stronger.

During that visit, Greg signed up for and attended a Rock Steady Boxing Level 1 class and said the 90-minute session was unlike anything he'd ever experienced before. Not only did he get a great workout, but hitting the heavy bag and the coaches' mitts as they called out punches enabled him to release some of the aggression he'd been feeling ever since he'd received his diagnosis. "It felt great to just hit something and hit it hard," he said.

After the session, Greg lingered to learn more about the program and was impressed by the level of fitness it promoted. He discovered that Rock Steady Boxing was not just a puncher's workout but a comprehensive program that included all of the physical exercise that those with Parkinson's need in order to achieve a healthy lifestyle. "My wife and I were extremely impressed with the positive attitude, camaraderie, and physical exercise involved," he said. "Right from that first class, I was hooked and wanted more, but the coaches told me it was only available in Indianapolis. I was disappointed, but they told me they wanted to expand and were hoping to get something started in New England, and they asked if I could help."

Upon returning to New Hampshire, Greg began reaching out to everyone he could think of in the Parkinson's community to tell them about Rock Steady Boxing. He e-mailed Parkinson's people in positions of authority in hopes of finding a similar type of program in his area, but there wasn't anything like it in New England. When he couldn't locate such a program, he tried to start one, but because Rock Steady Boxing was not well known on the East Coast, it proved to be a difficult concept to sell. He talked about the benefits of the program to those in his young-onset Parkinson's support group, and although they listened politely, Greg could tell they weren't interested. Frustrated and unsure of how to proceed, Greg returned to the YMCA and tried to forget about Rock Steady Boxing for the time being.

Fortunately for Greg, his wife did not forget what Greg had gotten out of his session in Indianapolis. That Christmas, she presented him with a Groupon for six private one-hour boxing lessons at a gym in Chelmsford, Massachusetts, where fighters Mickey Ward and Dickie Eklund trained. Greg was so nervous at the thought of training in a gym used by professional fighters that he waited six months before redeeming the gift certificate. When he finally came out of his corner and drove over to the gym, he had no idea he was about to meet the man who would change his life forever, boxing coach Albert Latulippe.

"I had no idea what I was getting myself into when I met Al," Greg said with a laugh. "But in the end, he became the older brother I never had."

At 6'3" and 275 pounds, Al, or "Big Al" as he is often called, was a physically intimidating presence, but the personal trainer and certified strength and conditioning coach was patient as Greg described his condition, the Rock Steady Boxing program, and how he wanted to emulate something like it for his own fitness routine. Al listened and then agreed to teach Greg basic boxing. Before long, he had Greg boxing three-minute rounds. "I had to stop along the way and rest because I was out of breath," Greg said. "We closed our session with the core exercises that are essential to boxing, but I could only do two or three push-ups and I couldn't complete a single sit-up—that's how out of shape I was."

Greg continued working out with Al, and before long, his physical fitness began to improve. His Parkinson's symptoms seemed to stay at bay after a session, and even the coach saw a difference in his client. Al began researching Rock Steady Boxing on his own and discovered there was a way to become an affiliate of the organization. He told Greg he thought the two of them should go to Indianapolis and take the training course to become certified Rock Steady Boxing coaches. Greg hesitated, but Al told him that he believed Greg, as someone with Parkinson's disease, could offer inspiration, hope, and help to other members of the community as a coach. Greg acquiesced, and the two made plans to travel to the Hoosier heartland in late summer.

Their wives were not as enthusiastic about the plan, both thinking the idea was more than a little mad—not the part about the guys becoming Rock Steady coaches, but the part where they were going to drive halfway across the country together. They had known each other for only eight weeks, for crying out loud! Why not give it some more time, get to know one another better, and then make the trip?

Timing could have been better, but the duo knew it was now or never. Although Greg was nursing a knee injury and Al's wife was seven months pregnant with their first child, the men were determined. They packed the car and headed for the highway.

Al and Greg arrived in Indianapolis on August 1, 2013, and drove over to the Rock Steady gym to get the lay of the land. Al had never seen a live session before and was fascinated by what he witnessed. Just by watching a class in progress, the two learned a lot about the program's philosophy, method, and results. Although the exercises are all geared to improve the strategic areas that affect Parkinson's disease, Al and Greg discovered it was not a one-size-fits-all proposition. Every boxer who comes to Rock Steady Boxing is evaluated and placed in one of four class levels, with exercises tailored to their specific needs. Each class is anchored with an appropriate number of coaches and "cornermen" (support givers) for the number of participants.

"What is so great about the program is that it can be modified if the person needs it to be," Greg said. "The participant may run the same drills, but they can change it if they need to. For example, you don't have to do a full squat to get the benefit if you have bad knees, and I have seen some fighters do wall push-ups if they can't get all the way down to the floor for the regular kind. The idea is to push them hard and get them to bend but not break."

Although the pair from New Hampshire was content to watch from the sidelines, the Rock Steady coaches insisted that they join in on the sessions. Al and Greg laughed because they were still in their street clothes and had just eaten lunch, but they gamely entered the ring to take part in the drills and exercises. "Boy, were we hurting afterward, but thankfully, neither of us needed the puke bucket," Greg said.

Al and Greg returned the following day for Training Camp and were put through two days of intense workouts. Not only did they learn boxing skills, techniques, and the specific ways the program affects Parkinson's, but on the second day, they were able to work with actual Rock Steady Boxing clients at the third and fourth levels (those with moderate to severe Parkinson's symptoms), which Greg found to be rewarding. As soon as Training Camp began, it was over and at the end of their training, Al and Greg participated in a small graduation ceremony in which they were officially recognized as certified Rock Steady Boxing Coaches.

"It was extremely meaningful for me as a person with Parkinson's disease to be named a certified coach. I had a few tears in my eyes as I left, and I promised the other Rock Steady Boxing coaches that we would get something started on the East Coast very soon," Greg said.

Fulfilling that promise would prove to be a bit of an uphill battle, however. Al and Greg returned to New England, continued their workouts at a gym in Lawrence, Massachusetts, and demonstrated the Rock Steady Boxing method whenever and wherever they could. Greg talked about the program constantly in his support group meetings, and although clients were not beating a path to the door, a few expressed interest, which gave the two the encouragement they needed to continue.

In October, 2013, Rock Steady Boxing (Indianapolis) was among the presenters at the World Parkinson's Congress in Montreal, Canada, and received a lot of positive feedback from those in attendance. As a start-up affiliate of the parent organization, Greg and Al benefitted from the response. They heard from a number of Parkinson's disease officials in Massachusetts and New Hampshire who had learned about the program at the event and wanted to know more about it. There was interest from the Massachusetts chapter of the American Parkinson's Disease Association (APDA), and Greg and Al even met with Renee LeVerrier, a person with Parkinson's disease who works with those who have movement disorders. Renee joined Al and Greg for a class, enjoyed the workout, and recommended it to others.

"Despite my attempt to live a yogic, peaceful approach to life, there are moments when I want to haul off and hit something. Hard. Maybe even several times … whether I am waiting on a dose of meds to kick in, fumbling to zip up my jacket … the *argh* moments of life with Parkinson's disease build up throughout the day. It's incredible how the frustration dissipates when I take it out on a punching bag," Renee wrote on a Parkinson's-related blog in January of 2014.

Although the endorsement was great, Greg said it was still a difficult time. He and Al had thought things would start to take off after that, but getting the program started still took a lot of time and a lot of hope.

Slowly but surely, people began to gravitate to the program and the Rock Steady Boxing Boston affiliate started attracting new recruits who liked the program and stuck with it. The media took notice as well. The *Lawrence Eagle-Tribune* ran a front-page article on the venture, and the *Boston Globe* did a feature piece as well. The local CBS and ABC affiliates aired short segments, which caused even more people to check out Rock Steady Boxing Boston—and a few even stayed!

In June 2014, almost a year after they started their journey, Al and Greg did a presentation in Concord, New

Hampshire, and had enough people interested in Rock Steady Boxing to start a second location. They attended the Partners for Parkinson's conference run by the Michael J. Fox Foundation and the pharmaceutical company AbbVie. Al was recognized by the media in conjunction with "Parkinson's Awareness Day" in April at the Massachusetts statehouse. "It seems that the more exposure we get, the better we become," Greg said.

Rock Steady Boxing Boston eventually relocated from its original gym to a new facility in Lawrence at the rejuvenated mill buildings known as the Riverwalk, and since the move, their number of boxers has more than doubled. The group applied for and received a grant from the National Parkinson's Foundation to create a new Rock Steady Boxing Boston program for the Beth Israel Deaconess Medical Center in conjunction with the Harvard Medical Group. The initial class accommodated 12 boxers and now has a waiting list of 40 people. Greg said they are up to 75 consistent boxers, field a constant stream of phone and e-mail inquiries about the program, thanks to the media coverage in recent months, and still try to take advantage of every opportunity that comes their way. "Things have just blown up for us. We had to add five classes to make room for everyone we could," Greg said.

Today, Greg is no longer the frustrated computer software engineer who once lamented his fate. Rock Steady Boxing and Al literally saved his life. Thanks to the program, he has a new lease on life. His blood work is the best it's ever been, his medications have not increased, and his doctors say he is doing great. Greg says others should look into the program because it offers people hope, camaraderie, and confidence.

"Parkinson's will steal your life if you let it, and while this is not a cure, this is what we've got," he said. "Rock Steady Boxing enables me to maintain a certain quality of life. I've lost weight. I'm stronger, and even my neurologist has noticed a positive change in me. At the end of the day, I may still have Parkinson's disease, but Parkinson's disease doesn't have me."

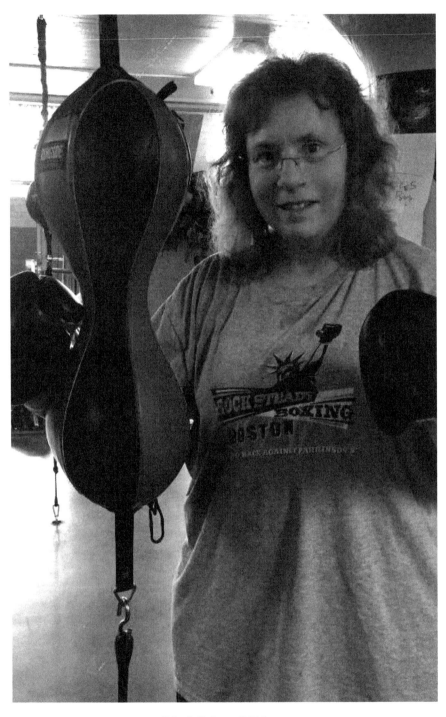

Madeleine O'Mara
Rock Steady Boxing Boston

ROUND 3

Breaking the Fall

"I made the most of my ability."
—Joe Louis

Every young person who has ever delivered newspapers around the neighborhood has a house that he or she dreads collecting from week after week. It is usually the home of an older person with a cantankerous attitude, someone who smells of mothballs or insists on paying the paper bill in small change. There is one on every route, and they tend to make the job more than a little unpleasant.

For Madeleine O'Mara of Amherst, New Hampshire, that customer was a woman who never answered the door with a smile. She greeted the young paper carrier with a muffled "hello" while her jaw bounced up and down like a needle in a sewing machine. Instinctively, Madeleine knew the woman was ill, but she could not imagine what affliction could cause such a spasm, and naturally, she was too polite to ask. Instead, she merely collected the money for the weekly delivery and went about her business wondering why the woman couldn't stop her mouth from going up and down and praying she would never end up like the woman. "What a foreboding thought that was," she said.

That was Madeleine's first experience with Parkinson's disease and it was a powerful one, but it would not be her last. Although she cannot remember at what point she made the connection between her customer's problem and the movement disorder, she does remember the moment when fate must have misheard her childhood wish: The day her neurologist told her she had young-onset Parkinson's disease and she realized she had become the very person she dreaded. "I guess something must not have translated correctly," she said.

In the early 1980s, Madeleine's paper-route days were far behind her. The happy, healthy twenty-something was fresh out of college, working as an electrical engineer at a computer company, and was quickly moving up the ranks. She was an amiable employee and a diligent worker who went above and beyond the call of duty whenever she could for the job she loved. She was also a well-rounded individual who spent her free time engaged in a wide range of physical activities including softball, basketball, and floor hockey; hikes through the White Mountains; and checking into the occasional aerobics class at her employer's on-site gym.

Madeleine was the last person anyone would suspect of having movement issues; however, one night in the late 1990s as she sat reading her newspaper, she suddenly felt the thin sheets quiver in her grip. She put the paper down and examined her hands but didn't notice them shaking. She excused the issue as a one-off event and promptly forgot about it. After all, she was far too young for it to signal a serious threat to her health, right?

In 2002, just shy of her 20th anniversary with her company, Madeleine was laid off. Although it was a blow, she wasn't one to stay down for long. Within three months, she was hired as a software engineer at a computer operating-system company. It was a different atmosphere than what she had been used to. At her old job, she had always been part of a team, but now she was an individual contributor. Still, she jumped at the opportunity to prove herself, and thanks to her exemplary work ethic, she was quickly promoted.

Madeleine had been at her new job for about two years when she began to experience a slight but visible tremor in her right leg, along with a twitching in her right thumb and forefinger. It wasn't affecting her work performance, so she let it go for more than a year. She might have let it go on even longer, but in the fall of 2005, she took the morning off work to attend her annual physical exam and her doctor noticed the tremor in her leg. He told her she needed to see a neurologist as soon as possible. Madeleine made the appointment for October and once again took a morning off from work. After conducting a routine examination, the specialist invited Madeleine into his office, where he delivered his diagnosis. "I was stunned, though not surprised," she said. "I had all of the classic symptoms of Parkinson's disease—small handwriting, unilateral tremor, and rigidity. Not only did my right arm not sway, it was so rigid that it was stuck bent at the elbow."

Throughout the drive back to the office, Madeleine's mind was filled with questions she didn't have answers for: Why her? How would this affect her life? Would it shorten her lifespan? Would she develop dementia? Prudently, she decided to seek a second opinion and, for the moment, keep her diagnosis to herself.

The second neurologist concurred with the original diagnosis and suggested that Madeleine might benefit from medication. She agreed, unaware of the roller-coaster ride she was in for. As she began what she calls "the unceasing and ever-changing dance with drugs," her first pharmaceutical cocktail helped decrease the severity of her tremors, but it increased the amount of daytime drowsiness she experienced.

Over the course of two years, Madeleine was involved in two auto accidents, veered off the road several times, and was stopped by the police on more than one occasion for erratic driving. Her sleep at night was also fragmented, which led to concentration difficulties and, eventually, problems at work. She endured the frustration of trying to type and involuntarily hitting the wrong key, as well as bouts of amnesia that resulted in her having no memory of hosting at least one meeting, and increased absenteeism. Although she still had not divulged her condition to anyone at her job, her manager alluded to the change in her productivity and sensed that something was wrong. Finally, the unthinkable happened: Madeleine received her first bad performance review. "That was more devastating than being told I had Parkinson's," she said. "Work was my life and I enjoyed it. Now I was despondent."

Madeleine knew she had to make a few changes. She decided to find a new neurologist, and she also decided that the time had come to tell her family about her condition. The timing was terrible because her mother was in a nursing home and quite ill and Madeleine had been caring for her stepfather, who was suffering with advancing Alzheimer's. She was apprehensive about making an announcement but knew that ongoing anxiety would only decrease her medication's effectiveness. But *how* to tell everyone was another question. Her family was small, so getting them together wouldn't be an issue, but she didn't know if she should do it in person. Should she call everyone individually? Arrange a conference call? Write a letter? Madeleine finally settled on making her announcement at a family dinner at her aunt's house. During a lull in the conversation, she said she needed the floor, and without preamble, she blurted the news about her diagnosis. "I didn't hear any reaction. I didn't see any reaction, either, but then again, my eyes were focused on the floor at the time. They asked several questions and I answered them, but that was it. It was finally over," she said.

With her secret out, Madeleine went about the business of finding a new neurologist who could create a plan of care that would meet her needs. She sought out a movement disorder specialist and scored an appointment with a doctor of substantial pedigree. The physician's office was a 45-minute drive from Madeleine's home, but Madeleine knew it was worth it to get the best possible care. Once again, her diagnosis was confirmed. She was scheduled for a neuropsychological exam to establish a cognitive baseline, and Madeleine and her doctor began their search for the elusive Holy Grail of medicinal concoctions. The doctor did give her one emphatic prescription before she left the office: Exercise was unequivocal.

After meeting with her new physician, Madeleine felt better about her treatment plan but was still conflicted about her job. The company she worked for had a sabbatical incentive plan in which those who had worked for the company for five years were entitled to a five-week paid sabbatical. It was 2007 and her turn for some time off, but instead of being overjoyed at the prospect of some much-needed downtime, Madeleine wasn't exactly looking forward to it. She had some serious soul searching to do and some big decisions to make. She really wanted to finish her last assignment and begin her sabbatical on a high note. She sensed some dissatisfaction from her manager and was afraid she might be terminated upon her return.

She took her work home but couldn't get much done because her cognitive processes were stunted and after a long day at the office, her brain was burned out. She was able to finish the assignment, but she didn't experience the sense of accomplishment that she had experienced when she'd completed things in the past. In the waning hours before her sabbatical began, she expected some childish banter and good-natured well wishes from her colleagues, but there were none. "My departure was silent and uneventful," she said.

Madeleine planned to visit the gym and get into a fitness routine during her time off, but getting there proved to be difficult. Not only was the gym a half hour from her home, but the route she needed to take to get there took her past her place of business, and she hated the thought of traveling by her office complex and not going in to work.

Although she didn't spend time doing any physical exercise during her leave of absence, Madeleine struggled through plenty of mental gymnastics. Her time off was consumed with research, dialogue, and fear. She made a list of the pros and cons for leaving work permanently and ultimately decided that it was in her best interest to do so. "My biggest regret was telling my manager I was leaving on disability over the phone and not putting on my 'big-girl panties' and telling him in person," she said.

Telling the boss she was leaving might have been difficult, but being a full-time Parkinson's fighter would have its challenges as well. Madeleine knew she had to get serious about exercise. Her specialist had been very clear about that, so Madeleine found a rehabilitation hospital that offered an eight-week Parkinson's disease exercise program and signed up for it. Classes were held twice a week and consisted primarily of stretches. Madeleine hadn't realized how badly her body had deteriorated in such a short time.

When someone has a condition such as Parkinson's, it's difficult to know if changes in the body are due to the illness, are side effects of the prescribed medication, or are merely effects of age, but Madeleine couldn't rise from a chair without using her arms, her gait was slow and unsteady, and she fell daily because her balance was poor. In the years since she had been diagnosed with Parkinson's, she'd also been told she had restless leg syndrome (RLS) and dystonia in her right foot. Both are painful neurological conditions. While RLS is characterized by a strange desire to move the lower limbs around and by uncomfortable feelings within the legs themselves, dystonia is a condition in which prolonged muscle contractions cause the afflicted body part to twist, repeat actions, or situate itself into an abnormal posture. In Madeleine's case, her foot dystonia caused the muscles that control her right foot to remain in a state of contraction. The sole of her foot faced her left leg, and her toes curled upward. "Nobody told me Parkinson's would be so painful," she said.

Madeleine attended the exercise class whenever it was offered, and it did help for a while. She learned to be conscientious of her stooped posture, her mobility improved, and she mastered the art of rising from a chair without using her arms. Then she plateaued. She needed to find something that would challenge her.

She first heard about the Rock Steady Boxing program through an imaging technician when she was in the x-ray lab for her annual mammogram. Madeleine offhandedly mentioned her Parkinson's diagnosis in casual conversation, and the tech told her she had a colleague whose husband was also a Parkinson's patient. The tech said he had found boxing to be extremely helpful both physically and from a therapeutic standpoint. Madeleine was intrigued to hear more. She knew a little about the sport from having attended Golden Gloves bouts with her father, and she was interested in learning more about how it could help with her Parkinson's.

The technician told her the name of the program, and when Madeleine went home, she immediately looked up the Rock Steady Boxing website. She clicked on the link that said "Find A Class Near You" and was directed to Rock Steady Boxing Boston. Madeleine was dismayed. Boston? She couldn't drive to Boston regularly when she lived in New Hampshire. She meandered through the website, watching videos of the classes, and when she returned to the Boston affiliate page, she noticed that the classes weren't in Boston at all but in Lawrence. Lawrence was an hour-long drive, but it was doable. She filled out the contact form and was told when and where to show up for her first session. The class was scheduled for March 27, 2014.

"When I got there, I met Al, who ran the class, as well as Greg, who had Parkinson's himself. I did well with the initial stretching, but my range of motion lacked," she said. This was especially apparent during her first Good Morning Stretch, in which participants sit on the floor with their legs extended in front of them with their arms extended above their heads. Al barked at everyone to get their arms up over their heads, but Madeleine couldn't do it. He made the request again. A third time, the order was directed specifically toward her.

"Madeleine, arms over your head!" He said.

Her arms were approximately shoulder high. "I told him this is as far as I could go," she said.

He nodded as if he understood and moved on. There were calisthenics, punching bags, and core exercises. Madeleine said it took all she had to accomplish three sit-ups. Afterward, Al asked her how she had liked her first Rock Steady Boxing session. She told him she loved it and couldn't wait to come back. "Hitting the bag was so cathartic," she said. "Who knew I could become a boxer?"

Madeleine became Rock Steady Boxing Boston's first regular client. Although Al and Greg were training three times a week, Madeleine started to come twice a week. In each class, she learned more about Al and Greg's own Rock Steady Boxing experience and how it had touched their lives. In a short time, she too was in the gym three times a week, giving every ounce of energy she had to each class. The trio became incredibly close: Madeleine was the new recruit, Greg was her comrade-in-arms, and Al served as the encouraging drill sergeant. When Madeleine had been in the program for a while, she was anointed with the Rock Steady

Boxing nickname "Stone," which not only made her a true member of the family but also cemented her place in Rock Steady Boxing Boston's foundation.

Not long after Madeleine joined the Rock Steady Boxing program, there was a period of frustration when no one new was coming in and word of the program didn't seem to be spreading. "We talked about being more proactive when word of mouth was not enough," she said. "We brainstormed new ideas, and that brainstorming session gave us a sense of empowerment. I volunteered to make a flyer. Al loved it and took over its final copy. We handed them out at Parkinson's events and in doctors' offices. Finally, our class began to grow. Greg and I kept improving. The dream was becoming a reality."

On her first-year anniversary in the Rock Steady Boxing program, there was no question that Madeleine was stronger and had better range of motion, better motivation, and better stamina. When she lost her balance in the past, she would fall. Thanks to the program, however, she now has the ability to catch herself. On those occasions when she does fall, she knows how to fall correctly in order to avoid injury. In addition to the physical benefit, Madeleine says the program gives her a wealth of intangibles, such as camaraderie, support, and a family unit that she never could have imagined.

During a checkup with her neurologist in 2015, the doctor commented that she looked great and there was no need to increase the dosage of her medication. The doctor has seen videos of Madeleine and Greg working out; she has begun recommending Rock Steady Boxing to other patients and keeps the program's literature in the office.

In August of 2015, Madeleine made the decision to travel to Indianapolis to become a certified Rock Steady Boxing coach. She not only wanted to be able to help Al with the newcomers but also really wanted to see the place and meet the people who inspired Al and Greg.

When she arrived in Indianapolis, Madeleine was amazed by the headquarters facility. They had everything! No space went unused! Classes were full, and she found the sounds of music, the impromptu dance, and the voices of encouragement exhilarating. "I can't say that the staff was 'working,' because it looked as though they were simply having fun doing what they love. They are ubiquitous, and they have my utmost respect. They are the present and the future of Parkinson's therapy."

Although it's been 10 years since Madeleine's diagnosis, it has been a lifetime since she was that earnest newspaper girl quivering in fear at the thought of developing a condition that could leave someone uncontrollably weak. Today, she continues to work out at Rock Steady Boxing three times a week and serves as a coach for a class.

"Thanks to Rock Steady Boxing, I am physically and mentally stronger than before," she says.

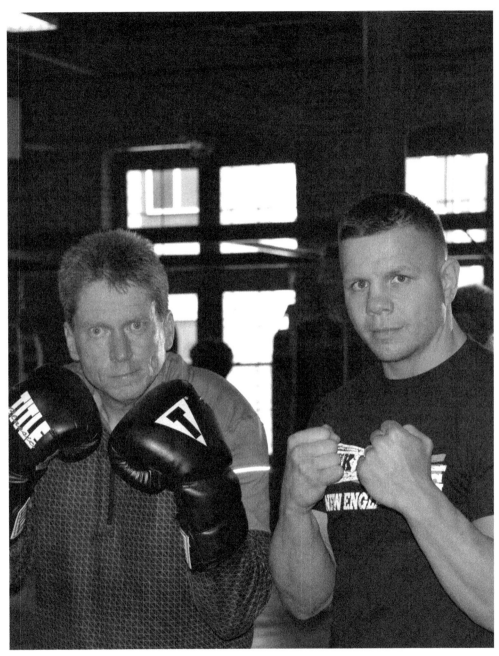

Michael Quaglia and Coach Rich Gingras
Rock Steady Boxing New England

ROUND 4

The Fight of My Life

"Never give up on yourself … no matter what."
—George Foreman

In September 2006, Michael Quaglia seemed to have it all. After spending most of his working life in his family's factory making molds and dies for corporate jewelry, he grew tired of merely getting by on his blue-collar income. He longed to find a position that would give his finances some wiggle room and enable him to be a better provider to his wife, Donna, and daughter, Carissa.

At the age of 37, he took a job as a headhunter in the highly competitive Boston area, where he spent his days networking with key contacts at area corporations, strengthening business relationships over power lunches and rounds of golf, and helping recruiters match engineering talent to the right company. Michael loved his new role, and the money wasn't bad either. Thanks to his success, the Quaglias were no longer living paycheck to paycheck but were living the American Dream. There was not only enough money to cover the bills but plenty left over to allow them to do all things they wanted to do but thought they could never afford. There were trips to Disney World, Kentucky, and the Florida Gulf Coast. Michael served as Carissa's softball coach and was present at other athletic events. He worked out a few times each week and even played a little poker on the side. "In my mind, I had made it in corporate America, and I was only 41 years old," he said.

By anyone's definition, it was a charmed life, and after five years with the company that had given him his start, Michael left his position in order to join a small start-up firm. The new job lasted only eight months, however.

Michael's previous employer was eager for him to rejoin the fold and made him an offer he couldn't refuse. "It was a great offer to return, so I did," he said. But there was something brewing below the surface—something that would tarnish the golden life the Quaglias were enjoying, would challenge Michael in ways he had never thought possible, and would nearly take him down for the count. The first indicator that there might be a problem had come when Michael was still toiling away in the family factory. He noticed his little finger shook uncontrollably whenever he bent it, but he didn't think anything about it until the day his whole hand shook when he leaned over to retrieve something from the floor. He also realized that over the years, his left shoulder had grown stiff and sore. Assuming he might have a routine rotator-cuff problem, he decided to bring up the issue at his next doctor's appointment.

The problem would prove to be anything but routine. After sharing his symptoms with his personal physician, Michael was referred to a neurologist who put him through a battery of tests and CAT scans to determine what was wrong. When nothing out of the ordinary appeared, he was sent to an orthopedist, who gave him a cortisone shot for his shoulder and sent him on his way. Three weeks later, Michael returned for his follow-up appointment; as the specialist examined his shoulder, he noticed the tremor in Michael's hand and a concerned look flashed across his face.

"He got up and wrote something on a piece of paper. It was the name of another neurologist. He called and set up an appointment for me, and even though I still didn't know what was wrong with me, I was starting to get very nervous," Michael said.

That nervousness turned to guttural fear when, just prior to his appointment with the new neurologist, Michael slipped and fell on the stairs of his house. Trembling, he told his wife it felt as if the whole left side of his body was dying. Donna held her husband and assured him that everything would be all right, but by this time, even she was beginning to have her doubts. Would they ever find out what was wrong?

A week later, a possible answer presented itself. As Michael and Donna got ready for their doctor's appointment, they saw Michael J. Fox on the *Today Show*. The *Family Ties* and *Back to the Future* star talked about his battle with Parkinson's and recalled some of his early experiences with the disease. The Quaglias could not believe what they were hearing. Fox's descriptions sounded exactly like what Michael was going through. They sat riveted to the screen, taking in each word, and when the segment was over, Michael looked at Donna. Donna looked back at Michael.

"It was then that we both knew," Michael said.

Of course, knowing something in your heart and having that suspicion confirmed by a medical professional are two different things. When the Quaglias arrived at the neurologist's office, they held on to the hope that the neurologist might offer another possible explanation for Michael's condition, but unfortunately, their instincts proved to be correct. After greeting the couple, reviewing Michael's medical history, and putting him through a series of exercises, the specialist blurted the bad news: Michael had Parkinson's.

To say that Michael and Donna were shocked would be an understatement. They were devastated by the pronouncement, momentarily stunned into silence. Michael eventually composed himself enough to ask what he could expect from his situation, and although he can no longer remember the doctor's name, he cannot forget what the man told him. "He said, 'Imagine how you are right now and multiply those symptoms by ten. That's what you will be like a decade from now.' I was then told to Google Parkinson's in order to find out more," Michael recalled.

Convinced he had only a few good years left, Michael turned to the Internet, but most of what he found left him angry and depressed. He flatly refused to return to the doctor who had diagnosed him and instead found a physician at a Boston hospital who had experience with young-onset patients. His name was Dr. David Simon. Michael called Dr. Simon's office to schedule a preliminary consultation but was chagrined to find out there was a six-month waiting list.

"As someone with a lot of sales experience, I know that in order to get the results you want, you have to talk to the person who makes the decisions," he said. "I found the doctor's e-mail address and contacted him directly. I had an appointment two weeks later."

The visit was a positive one. Michael's new physician not only gave him hope but also assured him that a Parkinson's diagnosis was not a death sentence. He took the time to educate Michael on the condition and told him stories of patients who had been battling Parkinson's for more than twenty years and were still living life to its fullest. The doctor shared the latest studies on Parkinson's and got Michael started on Azilect, a drug used to curb the shakiness associated with the disease. He also talked about the importance of exercise but never mentioned a specific fitness program. With so much information to wrap his brain around, Michael let that last piece of advice fall from his radar.

It was a fateful decision, but a common one. As Michael settled into his new role as a Parkinson's patient, he continued to carry on with his life as though nothing had changed. He took his medications religiously but made few lifestyle adjustment and paid little attention to his physical, emotional, or mental health. After seven years, the denial caused him to deteriorate. He tipped the scales at 230 pounds. His voice weakened. He had no arm movement, and his leg dragged behind him. Years of pent-up anxiety led to deep-seated depression, paranoia, insomnia, and isolation. He no longer went out to social events. He rarely communicated with anyone, and he began to experience problems at home and work. "I was going downhill," he said. "I wasn't me anymore."

Michael knew he needed to do something before it was too late, and one night in 2014 while searching the Internet, he came across a video produced by Purdue University highlighting a relatively new and unconventional exercise program designed to combat Parkinson's: Rock Steady Boxing. Michael watched the four-minute video repeatedly, and with each screening, he became increasingly convinced that this program could give him a new lease on life. He found a Rock Steady location sixty miles away and called the number listed on the website. He spoke to head coach Greg Geheb, whose passion for the program confirmed Michael's initial feeling of excitement and made him determined to bring Rock Steady Boxing to a gym near him.

In order to do that, however, Michael needed to learn the basics. He researched boxing clubs in his area and signed up for a free introductory class at Fight2Fitness, but when the night of his first session arrived, his nerves kicked in, he couldn't find his sneakers, and he nearly talked himself out of going. Realizing it was now or never, Michael grabbed an old pair of work boots and put them on, telling himself it didn't matter what he looked like.

"The first folks I met there were Christy Gibney and Ben Kiley, who helped out around the gym and ran a few classes. During my session, Christy began calling punch combinations and I attacked, releasing years of pent-up frustration. As a first-timer, I must have looked awkward, but I didn't care. It felt great," Michael said.

When class was over, a tired but happy Michael thanked Christy for the session and gave her the Rock Steady Boxing information he'd printed from the website. He asked her to give the information to the gym owner in hopes that the owner would call to find out more. Christy promised, and the next day, Michael received a call from Rich Gingras, who, unbeknownst to him, was not only the owner of Fight2Fitness but also a Golden Gloves champion and the star of the reality television series *The Contender*.

Rich told Michael he was a busy man but he had read over the information and wanted to help. The two set up an appointment to talk the next day, and when Michael arrived, Rich seemed unfazed by the involuntary muscle movements that caused Michael to sway back and forth. He ignored the jerky gestures and the way Michael stuttered when he talked. Rich merely asked about Michael's condition and why he thought boxing could make a difference. It was an in-depth conversation, and it wasn't long before the two clicked.

Rich took Michael under his wing and invited him to work out with his regular classes free of charge. He also became a very dear friend who was accepting of Michael's diagnosis and never made him feel uncomfortable about his symptoms. Once while the pair were in a restaurant, Michael began moving uncomfortably and was feeling self-conscious. Without missing a beat, Rich noticed the spasm and immediately started dancing and singing to pull focus from Michael and onto himself. "He put his arm around me and said, 'This is my friend, anyone have a problem with that?'" Michael remembered. (Naturally, no one in the dining room took up the challenge.) "He just has a way of helping people feel good about themselves."

As he worked with Michael, Rich also noted improvements in Michael's condition and watched videos about the Rock Steady Boxing philosophy. After two months of training together, both men were sold on the validity of this unique treatment program and decided the time had come to travel to the Midwest. "It was time to go to Indianapolis and become certified," Michael said.

When Michael and Rich traveled to Indianapolis, it was an emotional and inspiring experience to see Rock Steady Boxing in action. Michael not only came to grips with the reality of having an incurable disease but also knew that the professionals on staff could help teach him how to fight it. He also saw how the program was affecting Rich. Though Michael had known the professional fighter for only three months, he was moved to tears when he saw how emotionally invested Rich was.

After receiving certification, Michael and Rich opened up a Rock Steady Boxing affiliate in the Fight2Fitness gym in Pawtucket, Rhode Island, that provides encouragement and a tough-love approach to inspire maximum effort, speed, strength, balance, and flexibility. The program has been well received by the public, including Beth McCrae of Epoch Senior Living, who attended a class at Rock Steady Boxing New England with one of her residents, Nancy, who was going to her first boxing class. "The environment had great energy, and everyone was friendly. Nancy was immediately welcomed by people in her group … the workout was intense … the camaraderie was palpable … and they provide a great resource to those with Parkinson's in our community," McCrae wrote in a newspaper editorial.

Michael said none of his success would have been possible without the Rock Steady Boxing employees who have helped him along the way, including Kristy Follmar, Head Coach and Program Director, who, with her never-ending energy and positive support, is the first person to check in on everyone to make sure they are doing OK; Jessica Fithen, Affiliate Services Director, who is always available to answer questions; and Christine Timberlake, Coach and Member

Services, who lends her extensive knowledge to the program and makes it the best it can be. Michael also credits his wife, Donna, with being the rock who holds everything together for him and his daughter, Carissa, who inspires him with her drive, talent, and work ethic. "She makes me laugh when I need it, and she gives me the strength to keep moving forward," he said. "I want to be an active part of both of their lives for as long as possible, so I am going to continue to push the workouts."

Today, Michael says he is in the best shape of his life. He regularly endures two- and three-hour workouts to push himself as much as possible. He's lost nearly 40 pounds and improved most of his Parkinson's-related symptoms, though slowness of movement continues to be an issue. He said those who saw him two years ago cannot believe the transformation that has taken place.

"Those with Parkinson's disease owe it to themselves, their families, and their friends to check out the program and see if it's right for them," he said. "It's the best support group you will ever be part of, but you have to decide to do it. For me, being Rock Steady means I'm done obsessing about my condition and I'm giving it the fight of my life."

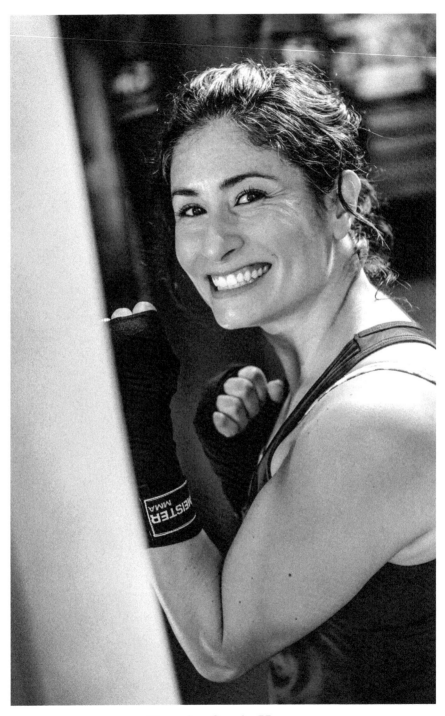

Veronica Garcia-Hayes
Rock Steady Boxing San Francisco

ROUND 5

Strong and Solid

"In boxing, you never know what is going to happen."
—Mickey Rourke

Dear Family and Friends,

I am writing you today to share some not-so-great news. Some of you know, others may suspect, and some of you may have no idea, so I have decided to finally spill the beans to clarify any misinformation. I have been struggling with some health issues over the past few years, and it is becoming increasingly difficult to hide my symptoms...

Veronica Garcia-Hayes was in the prime of her life. At the age of 39, she was a full-time real estate professional in the San Francisco Bay Area who spent her days culling through listings, meeting with clients, visiting properties, organizing open houses, and filing lots of paperwork. She was also an avid hiker, runner, and cyclist who worked out regularly, participated in marathons, and even completed the

San Francisco AIDS Cycle, a seven-day, 545-mile ride to Los Angeles.

She was the kind of person whose weekends were always booked with things to do, places to go, and people to see. If she wasn't making extra money catering parties or tending bar with her friends occasionally, she might be visiting her large family or traveling with her husband, Dylan. "I guess you could say that we were a busy, social, active, and child-free couple," she said.

But all of that was about to change. In August 2009, Veronica and Dylan drove to Sonoma, California, for her mother-in-law's birthday celebration, and over a family dinner at a local restaurant, Veronica noticed that she could not open her left hand completely without forcing it. She assumed she must have pinched a nerve during one of her many activities, causing the hand to cramp, and she put it out of her mind for the time being and went on with evening's festivities. When she returned home, though, she called her mother, Barbara, and told her about the strange episode.

Barbara confessed that she had seen it in Veronica before. Over the past few months, she'd noticed a slight tremor in her daughter's hand, but she didn't know what to make of it, either. She had wondered if Veronica was merely tired from work or was a little hung over at times and didn't want to embarrass Veronica by asking her about it.

Veronica laughed at her mother's terrible joke and assured her that she did not have a problem with alcohol. After discussing it for a while, the two women agreed that Veronica should take up the problem with her personal physician at the next available opportunity, but before

Veronica could book the appointment, she received some wonderful news. She was pregnant. "Needless to say, I soon forgot all about what was happening to my left hand," she said.

She wouldn't be able to forget about it for long, though. As Veronica and Dylan began preparing for parenthood in those early months, the strange symptoms on her left side intensified. She took the issue to her general practitioner, but because of her condition, the doctor thought it best that she see a neurologist. She was referred to Dr. Rimma Ash of Kaiser, California, who asked a few questions, conducted a routine physical exam, and then ordered an MRI—a test that could have significant ramifications for the unborn child.

Although Veronica wanted to know what was going on, she didn't want to subject her baby to anything dangerous. The specialist understood and said that to achieve the necessary image without compromising the baby, only Veronica's head, neck, and chest would enter the scanning device while the rest of her body stayed outside of the machine and away from the strong magnetic field.

The results were somewhat vague. Veronica noted something that looked like white specks on her brain but didn't know what, if anything, they might be. The neurologist recommended she see a movement disorder specialist as soon as possible and referred her to Dr. Robin Fross in Hayward, California.

On November 24, the day before Thanksgiving, Veronica drove herself to her appointment without any fear about what she might hear. She had no idea what the doctors could be looking for, but she reasoned it couldn't be anything too serious. When Dr. Fross opened the door and saw Veronica sitting solo in the waiting room, the doctor's face fell. "Oh, you came alone," she commented.

"My heart sank," Veronica recalled. "I knew she was going to deliver bad news."

Dr. Fross led Veronica into her office, where she conducted yet another physical exam and went over the MRI results before delivering her verdict. "I believe you have early-onset Parkinson's disease," she pronounced.

Parkinson's. The word circled in Veronica's brain, but she couldn't grasp its meaning. As Dr. Fross patiently explained the condition and its symptoms, the terms and definitions went by her in a blur. As if to add insult to injury, when the specialist handed her some Parkinson's literature to take home and read at her leisure, Veronica was horrified to see so many older people staring at her from the brochures. *This isn't me*, she thought. *This can't be me!*

Dr. Fross promised to follow up with her soon, and when the consultation was over, Veronica walked slowly to her car. She tried to digest everything she had heard, but it was still such a haze. She reached for her phone and called her mother, but she burst into tears before she could get a single word out about the visit. Her mind was racing with questions that weren't covered in *What to Expect When You're Expecting*—questions such as *What do you do when you find out you have Parkinson's disease? How do you tell your husband? Should you drive yourself home in your condition? What would her life be like now?*

Veronica knew next to nothing about Parkinson's. No one in her family had it, but she did remember the names of a few famous people associated with the condition and took some comfort in the fact that they were alive. *OK, so I am not going to die*, she admitted to herself. *But how am I going to live with this? What does this mean for my baby and me?*

Although pregnancy and Parkinson's is not common, it's not unheard of, either. Because so few of these cases are reported, researchers have written very little on the subject. The data that has been collected is typically divided into one of two categories: the effect pregnancy has on Parkinson's disease and the effect Parkinson's disease has on pregnancy.

According to Dr. Susan M. Rubin, MD, Clinical Instructor and Director of the Women's Neurology Center at Glenbrook Hospital in Glenview, Illinois, although there can be an increase in both non-motor and motor Parkinson's symptoms during pregnancy, the increase is usually insignificant to the mother's overall health. Non-motor symptoms such as fatigue, mood swings, and constipation issues generally improve after delivery, but the progression of motor symptoms, including rigidity, shakiness, and slowed movement, tends to continue.

The biggest concern for Parkinson's patients who are pregnant is the possible birth defects that can result from antiparkinson medications. "The dopamine agonists, bromocriptine and pergolide (Permax) are considered relatively safe during pregnancy, but make it impossible to breastfeed because they block milk production," she said in her article "Parkinson's Disease in Women" for the American Parkinson Disease Association. "The remainder of the antiparkinson's medications carries a category C rating, meaning that animal studies suggest some risk but human studies are not available or have not confirmed that risk."

Because Veronica's Parkinson's symptoms were not affecting her daily life, she did not start taking any medication right away. In fact, for the majority of her pregnancy, she was more or less able to put her diagnosis on the back burner to concentrate on delivering a healthy child. Her feelings on the subject were a little harder to hide, however, especially when her pregnancy hormones kicked into high gear. She said whenever she started feeling sorry for herself, she would go out to the car and cry or take solace in a shower, where she could let the tears fall freely in private.

"I never denied my condition, but I didn't want to upset my husband," she said. "Even today whenever I get really angry, sometimes I just allow myself to be sad. Of course on other days, I tell myself to shut up and that life could be worse. Some days I just accept it, and some days, I can't believe this is my life. Luckily, on most days, I feel pretty good."

For reasons unrelated to Parkinson's, Veronica's pregnancy was considered high risk, but at 35 weeks, she gave birth to a beautiful baby girl whom she named Isa. Isa was early, but she was perfect, and over the next two years, Veronica focused solely on motherhood. She put Parkinson's in a corner and concentrated on her daughter's health and happiness. Her symptoms worsened during that time, however. Her balance was off. Her gait was off. Typing became difficult. She had trouble scrambling an egg, brushing her teeth, and dancing. She eventually had to face the music and focus her attention on herself.

As a proponent of holistic medicine, Veronica sought the help of a naturopathic doctor, someone who promotes wellness, prevents illness, and treats diseases using a wide array of natural and clinical methods. This doctor, Sergio Azzolino, suggested that she be tested for Lyme disease, a condition whose symptoms can mimic those of Parkinson's. He wanted to make sure Veronica had not been misdiagnosed.

"I hoped I had been misdiagnosed," Veronica said. "I was willing to try anything, and I left no rock unturned. I wanted to make sure I did my due diligence. My husband and I had traveled a lot. We backpacked and camped in many places, so I could have been exposed to anything."

Veronica tested positively for the bacteria and was treated for it, and for a period of time, she followed a natural approach to managing her symptoms while still seeing her neurologist. Her diagnosis remained unchanged, however, and in 2013, she realized the time had come to begin medication.

> *… I have put off taking medications, as they will not halt the progression of the disease but merely mask the symptoms. In addition, if the current medications work for me, they are only effective for a limited time period …*

Like many Parkinson's patients, Veronica had a trial-and-error period of finding the right medication to help with her symptoms. During this period, the doctors told her to keep doing whatever physical activity felt good, but they never offered any specific suggestions for exercise. Veronica reached out to a personal trainer who had helped one of her friends battling multiple sclerosis, so she could continue with her workouts, but little by little, movement in general became more difficult. "The medication I was taking just wasn't working for me," she said. "In 2014, I began levodopa therapy to regain command of my movements, and that's when I began to box."

Veronica's journey to Rock Steady Boxing San Francisco happened almost by accident. While attending a friend's party, she made the acquaintance of Simon Redmond, owner of Polk Street Gym, home to San Francisco's Rock Steady Boxing affiliate. Simon recognized Veronica's symptoms, and after the party, he tactfully asked their friend if it would be OK to contact her directly so he could tell her about their program.

Veronica was surprised to get the call. She hadn't realized her condition had become that obvious, but she was happy that Simon had thought of her. Her father and uncles had all been amateur boxers in their youth. Her grandfather was always a big fan of the sport, too, and having grown up watching matches alongside her family members, Veronica was excited at the prospect of stepping into the ring herself.

"I started boxing twice a week, and in no time at all, I was hooked," she said. "It's not easy, though. It works all parts of your body and brain. You have to move your hands and feet, keep your balance, maintain your speed, and think about your strategy. I love it so much, I wish I could box for real!"

Although she thought she was in great shape before her diagnosis, Veronica says Rock Steady Boxing San Francisco has brought her to a whole new level of fitness. Between her medication, weight training, yoga, and workouts at the Rock Steady Boxing gym, she is in the best shape of her life. There is no shortage of workouts at Rock Steady, and every day offers something different. Luckily, Veronica enjoys it all. Her favorite routine is hitting mitts with her coach, a cathartic workout that tends to be a favorite among Rock Steady Boxing clients, but she also enjoys working on the heavy bag and speed bag, and doing the double-end-bag drills. Veronica says that a typical day at Rock Steady Boxing might include aerobic exercises such as jumping jacks, hula-hoop, jump rope, footwork drills, and coordination routines. There are also targeted exercises such as push-ups, tricep dips, and core work.

"We learn how to walk. We learn how to fall, and there are even group exercises like tossing a ball to each other while jogging around!" Veronica said. "The variety of workouts is wonderful. The camaraderie is irreplaceable, and my arms look great! All kidding aside, it is probably one of the most comprehensive workouts for all ability levels and all stages of Parkinson's disease. It really is for everyone!"

Veronica said all of the Rock Steady Boxing coaches are wonderful people who bring something different to the table and that people with Parkinson's who visit the San Francisco gym will be treated to a great mix of folks who expect the most from their boxers. "I am especially grateful to Simon for contacting me and Coach Kim Woolley for not being a softy on us and treating us like she would any other client. That's all we really want."

Today, Veronica continues to work part time, going above and beyond on the days she feels great, and taking it easy on the days she is physically impaired. Her daughter is now a thriving six-year-old who loves to watch Veronica box and is a frequent visitor to the Rock Steady Boxing San Francisco gym. Isa can be found mimicking her mother's workouts on the heavy bag in the garage, sparring with her grandpa, and doing some yoga moves. Veronica says she knows her daughter will grow up to be fit and healthy because she has so many good examples in front of her. "Our family's fitness regimen is more like a lifestyle now," she says.

After all the years of running and biking for other causes; Veronica says it does feel weird to have the shoe on the other foot. She said although she may have more strength overall, she still battles with fatigue but has made peace with what she can and cannot do. Although it may take a little longer to recover from her workouts now than before Parkinson's, she knows that in the long term, it's well worth it. She is strong and solid, and with Rock Steady Boxing behind her, she's not going anywhere without a fight.

… It is true that I am different. Life is definitely more challenging. However, I need to feel as normal as possible. … Love, hugs, and kisses are welcome, (but) pity is not allowed. … I am Rock Steady.

Love,
Veronica

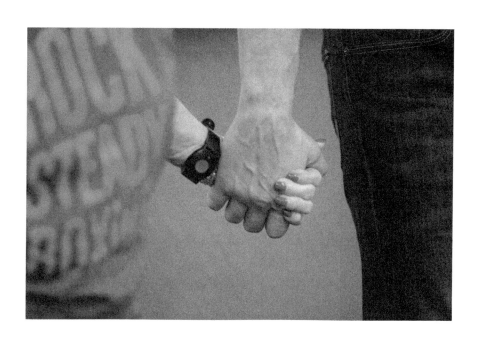

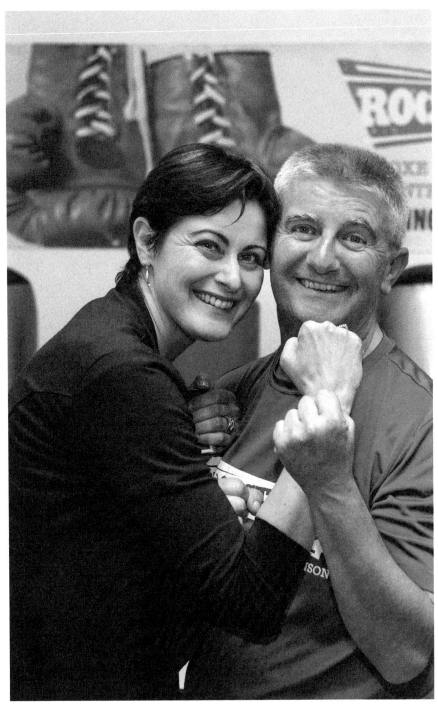

Paola Roncareggi and Tiberio Roda
Rock Steady Boxing Lake Como

ROUND 6

The Italian Stallion

"In the ring, I never really knew fear."
—Rocky Marciano

The Rock Steady Boxing program is not limited to individuals living in the United States. As word of the program and its benefits spread, it generated interest from the international community, who were eager to try it for themselves. Today, in addition to affiliates throughout the United States, the Rock Steady Boxing program has taken root in Canada, Australia, and even Italy, where 300,000 men and women are afflicted with Parkinson's disease. Tiberio Roda is one of them.

The province of Como is one of the most popular tourist destinations in northern Italy. Located in the Lombardy region and adjacent to Lake Como and the Alps, it is home to a number of churches, museums, theaters, parks, and palaces. It is also where Tiberio spends his days overseeing operations at Trafilerie San Paolo SRL, a steel-coil manufacturing firm in the small municipality of Erba, 25 miles north of Milan.

"Since 1966 we have offered our clients the highest-quality solutions for the improvement of cold-deformation technologies," Tiberio said. "Our customers are manufacturers who specialize in pressed hardware and use our products to create low-resistance bolts, nuts, and self-threading screws as well as low-, medium-, and high-resistance connecting parts."

The life of a business owner is a lot of things, but it is never dull. When Tiberio was not on the production floor ensuring that his products were made to exact specifications, he could be found studying spreadsheets, meeting with clients, and reviewing the latest research and developments in his industry. His home life was equally active. Although his two children were in their twenties and already out of the nest, Tiberio kept busy with the love of his life, Paola Roncareggi, working in his garden, going to cultural activities, enjoying his 3-D-printing hobby, and following myriad sports. "I enjoy snow skiing, sailboating and hang gliding; however, between 1995 and 2013, I did not do much in the way of exercise," he said.

Tiberio's first Parkinson's-related incident occurred in 2012 when he lost his balance and fell down a set of stairs, severely injuring his left side. Although he recovered from the accident, he noticed a persistent limp in his left leg as well as tremors that would not abate. In addition, he lost his sense of smell. His symptoms were not terrible and did not prevent him from keeping up with his duties at the office, but after a year, he decided to see a doctor about his condition. He wondered if it might be a lumbar spine problem or something related, but in July 2013, the 58-year-old was diagnosed with Parkinson's disease.

Naturally, the news came as a surprise, but Tiberio wasn't afraid of his doctor's words. In fact, he told his neurologist that if Parkinson's disease was a race, it was a race he intended to win. He knew very little about the condition aside from the tremors commonly associated with it, and when he went home, he scoured the Internet for additional information. "I didn't have any grief about my diagnosis— no denial, depression, or bad thoughts of any kind," he said. "My condition was stable enough that I did not have to start taking medications right away except for mucuna pruriens, an organic powder that comes from a specific type of Indian bean. For the most part, I accepted Parkinson's for what it was and began to fight back."

Tiberio's doctor told him that exercise was the key to maintaining control over his body, and over the summer holiday, Tiberio took long walks and intense hikes through the mountains. The fresh air and movement felt great at the time, but when he returned to his office in September, the reduction in activity caused his symptoms to reappear. Even more alarming, they were a little worse.

Tiberio turned back to the Internet in hopes of finding some suggestions, and that's when he found Rock Steady Boxing. As he navigated the organization's webpage and watched a video presentation about the program at the World Parkinson's Conference in Montreal, he wondered if a boxing regimen might be right for him. He wasted no time in finding out.

Tiberio joined the Palestra New Millenium (New Millenium Gym) under the direction of Enrico Milazzo and began to learn some of the basics of boxing. After experimenting with the boxing techniques for three months, he saw significant improvement in his symptoms and was determined to learn more. "I was very enthusiastic about boxing, and I wanted to find out more about this amazing program," he said.

He contacted the Rock Steady Boxing headquarters in Indianapolis and said that he wanted to bring the program to the European community. In January 2014, Tiberio traveled to the United States to become a certified Rock Steady Boxing coach.

"Love was in the air at the Rock Steady Boxing headquarters in Indianapolis," he said. "Everyone there was warm, welcoming, and it was easy to see the passion they have for what they do there. I trained alongside a group of boxing professionals, doctors, chiropractors, neurologists, and researchers who formed the first group of students for 2014."

When Tiberio returned to Erba, Paola couldn't help seeing a continued improvement in Tiberio's condition. After 22 years as a semiprofessional volleyball player, she became intrigued by the effect that sports could have in the healing process. That summer, she too traveled to Indiana to become a Rock Steady Boxing coach.

Now that they both had their coaching credentials, Tiberio and Paola were excited to help other people in Italy who had Parkinson's fight back against their diagnosis. In September 2014, the pair offered their first class. Within a few months, word about the program and its results spread, and in January 2015, the city of Logone al Segrino offered up a municipal gymnasium to serve as a Rock Steady Boxing rehabilitation center.

Tiberio and Paola were excited to have a home for their venture, but getting it up and running quickly was easier said than done. Thanks to logistical support from Milazzo's gyms in Ponte Lambro and Cesano Maderno, as well as crowd funding efforts for new equipment, they officially opened on March 18, 2015. The grand opening was attended by Antonio Rossi, Councillor for Sports in Lombardy, as well as one of the giants in Italian boxing, 1960 Olympic gold medalist and then middleweight world champion Nino Benvenuti. "I hope this is a new season for boxing, which for me is the most beautiful sport in the world. ... After the boom of the '50s and '60s ... boxing has experienced difficult times, but it has never disappeared even though it is a sport that asks a lot," Nino said at the opening. "You don't just commit, you have to grit your teeth and give everything only to discover that with tenacity you can go beyond your limits."

Tiberio and Paola christened their new venture Rock Steady Boxing Lake Como to reflect the beauty and charm of the area, and they worked hard to ensure that they have the support of the local medical and sports community. They partnered with Dr. Luca Morelli of the Centro San Fedele in Longone al Segrino, who is a former assistant professor at the Department of Physiology, School of Medicine, University of Pennsylvania, Philadelphia. He and his staff provide medical support and physiotherapy to the Rock Steady Boxing fighters, and through this partnership, Dr. Luca and Rock Steady Boxing have launched a study tracking the results of those who participate in the Rock Steady Boxing Lake Como program.

"Ours is the first gym of its kind in Europe and is managed by two certified trainers, assisted by a multidisciplinary medical center and supported by an FPI (Italian Boxing Federation) champion," said Tiberio. That champion is none other than Vincenzo Cantatore, the former European Light Heavyweight champion from Santo Spirito, Italy, who boasted a career record of 33 wins (27 by knockout), 5 losses, and 1 draw. After leaving the professional ring, Vincenzo spent his time developing a noncontact boxing program designed to help rehabilitate prisoners, hospitalized children, and young people with mental disorders.

Tiberio met Vincenzo in Milan at one of the many workshops that the boxer presented throughout the country. The two had an immediate connection. Vincenzo was intrigued with the Rock Steady Boxing method and readily agreed to help promote it in a variety of ways. He uses his vast social network and notoriety to spread the word about Tiberio's program and has even spoken about it on Radiotelevisione Italia (RAI), the Italian public broadcasting station.

The concept of Rock Steady Boxing, with Vincenzo's charitable endeavors, has garnered the attention and support of a number of many important and influential people throughout Italy. One of their biggest cheerleaders is Pope Francis himself. In April 2015, the pontiff met and spoke with Vincenzo after a general audience and expressed enthusiasm for the programs. Not only was one of his predecessors, St. Pope John Paul II, diagnosed with Parkinson's disease in 1991, making the condition near and dear to his heart, but he also applauds the fact that these programs are low- to no-cost and have the ability to reach many.

"Pope Francis is very popular here, and for me to know that he's approved our work is a boost to go straight on with our mission," Tiberio said. "I have a feeling that Pope John Paul II would have approved of mine and Vincenzo's work as well, if he would have known about Rock Steady Boxing before he died."

Although papal approval is no small accomplishment, for Tiberio and Paola, the biggest satisfaction comes from knowing that they have helped others fight back against Parkinson's. As more people hear about the Rock Steady Boxing program, there is more opportunity for the Lake Como affiliate to grow in the future. Tiberio says one of his boxers, a 47-year-old Parkinson's patient, will soon travel to Indianapolis to take the certification course and that he hopes more will follow in the months ahead.

"I've already had requests from a number of cities, including Turin, Venice, Rome, and Lecce, and we are putting together the numbers to see if we can make something happen in these areas," he said. "We are also working with the Italian Young Parkinson's Association as well as the boxer-writer Wilson Basetta, who is including a chapter on Rock Steady Boxing in his new book, and we hope to organize a noncontact Italian championship so that those with Parkinson's can compete and have fun with all that they have learned."

That is all in the future, however; at present, Tiberio has more than enough on his hands. In the middle of 2015, he and his brothers optioned to buy out the Trafilerie San Paolo factory, which created additional duties and demands in the workplace. Not long after that, the municipality of Longone al Segrino, which originally donated a local gymnasium to the Lake Como affiliate, announced that it would begin charging rent for the space. The amount was more than Tiberio and Paola were prepared to pay, forcing them to move.

Tiberio said that he keeps his fingers crossed that eventually there will be a cure for Parkinson's, but in the meantime, he's not giving up hope. "It's great to be part of the Rock Steady Boxing program. I am part of an advanced team fighting against Parkinson's disease, and we are going to knock it out."

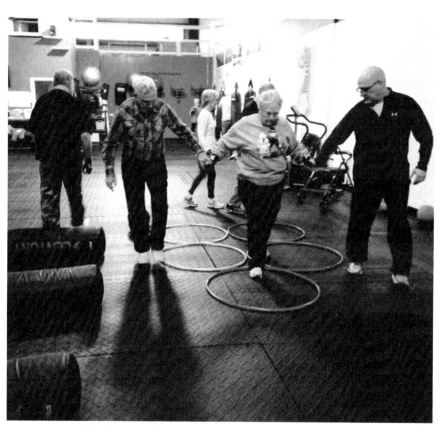

Rock Steady Boxing Brownsburg, Indiana

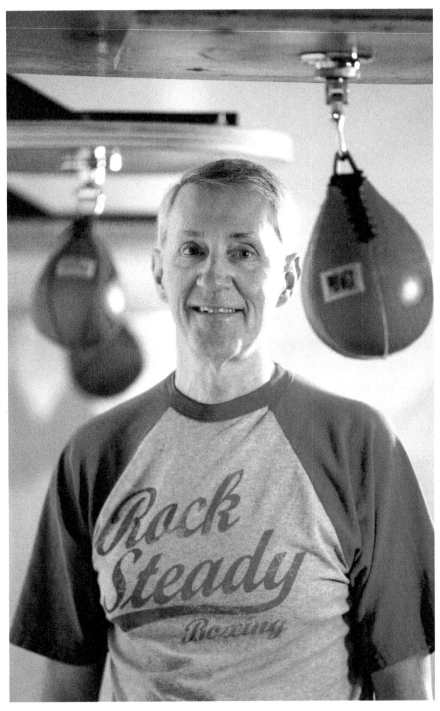

David Layman
Rock Steady Boxing Indianapolis

ROUND 7

Practice What You Preach

"Serving others is the price you pay for your room here on Earth."
—Muhammad Ali

David Layman has had more than his fair share of experience with Parkinson's disease over the years. As a Presbyterian pastor, he called on persons afflicted with the condition and felt a great deal of empathy for those whose speech had become so weak that it was hard for others to understand them, as well as those whose bodies trembled beyond their control. Although he was grateful for the opportunity to meet with them, pray for them, and share words of encouragement and hope, he had no intention of ever becoming one of them. "I never wanted to be on the other end of that empathetic glance," he said. "I never planned on becoming an object of pity."

The son of a Presbyterian pastor himself, David was born in Richmond, Indiana, but grew up in various locations throughout the Midwest. He studied at Carroll College in Waukesha, Wisconsin, before following God's call to the Louisville Presbyterian Theological Seminary in Kentucky and Yale Divinity School. After completing his studies, however, David longed to return to his roots. He remembered how fondly his parents had spoken about his hometown, and when he was offered a post at Richmond's Second Presbyterian Church in 1975, he jumped at the chance to take it.

His initial stint at home was a short one. After five years, David relocated to Greenville, Ohio, but returned to Richmond in 1988. This time, he was to lead the flock at First Presbyterian. During his second pastorate in Richmond, Second and then Earlham Heights Presbyterian merged with First. David was not only happy to be back home again in Indiana but also delighted to see old and new friends come together.

Throughout his nearly 40-year ministry, David was the kind of pastor who practiced what he preached. Many people throughout the community benefitted from his leadership on those issues that were important to him, such as drug and alcohol abuse, affordable housing, and healthcare. He was a founding member of Richmond's Habitat for Humanity chapter as well as of Hope House, a rehabilitation and recovery center for the homeless and for addicted men. He served many hours for these causes and also was a community member on Reid Hospital committees. In these areas and others, David worked tirelessly to extend his church's outreach ministry.

At the age of 60, David said, he began feeling the first stirrings of Parkinson's. He developed a tremor in his right hand that made writing sermons, composing e-mails, and using a computer mouse difficult. It was not uncommon for him to erase something he had previously written, press the wrong key, or click on an advertisement he didn't want to see. Before long, everyday tasks became problematic as well. He took longer to button his shirt each morning. He had trouble keeping food on his fork, which made him self-conscious about eating in public, and his increasingly wobbly handwriting became harder to read.

Eventually, David began to see the tremor as an occupational hazard. Having gotten to the point in his ministry where he no longer stood behind the pulpit to deliver the Sunday message, David preferred the intimacy of preaching near the congregation using a clip-on microphone and notecards to help him get through his sermon, but his hand shook so badly, he not only had trouble reading what he had written but also struggled to hang on to the cards.

"Graveside services were the worst," he said. "Without a podium to hold on to, my hand trembled uncontrollably and I worried that everyone was watching me shake instead of concentrating on the comforting words."

David tried to conceal his condition from those around him and downplayed its severity in his own mind. He kept his hand in his pocket whenever possible, and when dining in public could not be avoided, he ordered sandwiches, which could be eaten with two hands. When he caught a glimpse of himself in the video of his youngest daughter's wedding, however, he could no longer deny the truth. Something was seriously wrong. "I was shocked by what I saw and how pronounced the tremor was," he said. "I thought, *Who is this old, quivering guy walking my daughter down the aisle?* When I saw that footage, I knew I was only fooling myself."

David turned to his personal physician in hopes of getting to the bottom of the problem. The doctor examined him and prescribed an anti-tremor medication, but it failed to alleviate his symptoms. Next, David consulted with a neurologist, who diagnosed him with an essential tremor—a relatively common nervous disorder characterized by rhythmic shaking. The specialist recommended other types of medication in hopes of getting the tremor under control, but three years and several prescriptions later, David's condition continued to deteriorate. "It was very frustrating," he said.

David returned to his primary care physician, who suggested he seek a second opinion in Indianapolis. David agreed and made an appointment with Dr. Sarah Elizabeth Zauber at the Indiana University Neurology Center. Dr. Zauber is a neurologist who specializes in the treatment of movement disorders, deep brain stimulation, Parkinson's disease, dystonia, tremor, and more. Originally told there would be a four-month wait to see the esteemed physician, David was ecstatic when her office called to tell him there had been a cancellation and his appointment had been bumped up. David traveled the 75 miles from his home in Richmond to Indianapolis, where he was put through a barrage of tests similar to those he had endured before. When Dr. Zauber finished her assessment, she asked him if he would be surprised to learn that he had Parkinson's disease.

David was surprised, but the pronouncement didn't strike him as bad news at first. He realized that he had been misdiagnosed in the past and that perhaps the misdiagnosis explained why none of the medications worked. There was also some satisfaction in having a well-known condition shared by celebrity A-listers such as Michael J. Fox and Muhammad Ali. "There is some status in being able to say, 'I have Parkinson's disease,'" he said. "It sounds like a more significant challenge than an essential tremor. People have at least heard of it, and it puts you in some very good company. I may not be able to act like Fox or fight like Ali, but through this diagnosis, I actually have something in common with them. Who knew?"

Although he initially took the news in stride, when the dust settled and reality kicked in, David was less than enthusiastic about his prognosis. He had several questions. What did it mean to have a condition with no known cure? Could he die from it? What caused it to happen in the first place? He'd had heart bypass surgery several years before. Did that have something to do with it?

Dr. Zauber assured him that the bypass surgery didn't have anything to do with his Parkinson's and that in all likelihood, he would probably die from something other than Parkinson's, but David was not comforted. He thought back on all of the Parkinson's patients he'd met in the past and wondered if this was to be his future. Would he too have to endure increasing limitations over a long period of time? It was one thing to counsel others who were suffering and to encourage them to remain strong in the face of their challenges, but quite another to bear witness to it himself. Would he be able to walk the walk after years of talking the talk?

Dr. Zauber discussed David's condition with him at length and stressed the importance of exercise in helping him to remain strong in the face of his diagnosis. She told him about Rock Steady Boxing and how it was showing promise in helping folks delay or diminish the symptoms of Parkinson's. It was headquartered in Indianapolis. David thanked her for the suggestion, but a 75-mile drive seemed like a long commute for a workout. He played basketball at the local senior center to stay active, and although he had no qualms about intense physical exercise, he was never drawn to the sport of boxing. "As a pastor, I've always tried to encourage others to reason with each other and love one another, not step outside and fight it out," he said. "Besides, I have kind of a slender build and frame, so I am the last person you'd expect to see in a boxing ring."

When Reid Hospital announced that it was starting a Rock Steady Boxing affiliate program at its rehabilitation center, however, David decided to give it a try. He was among a group of six who showed up for class on that first day, and he immediately fell in love with the program. He liked the way Rock Steady Boxing blended traditional calisthenics with various boxing techniques. He liked the way the coaches pushed each participant to do his or her best without sounding like overbearing drill sergeants. Best of all, he liked being around other "Parkies," who understood the trials and tribulations he was going through.

Although Parkinson's affects between 7 and 10 million people worldwide, diagnosis is often the first experience most people have with the condition and its unique symptoms. David says it's easy to see why so many people who are diagnosed fall into a state of depression and self-pity as they contemplate the road ahead. They may feel some embarrassment about their tremors or other Parkinson's-related issues and may isolate themselves from their friends and family. This behavior only makes a bad situation worse and can create a vicious cycle that is not easy to overcome.

At Rock Steady Boxing, however, people with Parkinson's learn that they are not the only person in the world suffering with this condition, and that there is something they can do to fight back and they don't have to fight alone. Within the gym walls is a ready-made group of friends struggling to overcome the same challenges and ready to commiserate with a handshake, hug, or sympathetic eye roll (reserved mainly for those moments when a coach introduces something new).

"At Rock Steady Boxing, we are the majority and the coaches are in the minority!" David said.

David isn't sure why Rock Steady is so effective in combatting the symptoms of his disease, but he suspects it is a combination of things. He thinks that the forceful exercises may help the brain produce a little extra dopamine in the same way that rolling up the tube can help squeeze a little extra toothpaste onto the brush. As a proponent of holistic medicine and faith-based healing, he also feels attitude has something to do with it. David says whenever people believe they can improve, they have a better-than-average chance of succeeding.

Rock Steady Boxing benefits not only those people afflicted with Parkinson's disease but also their family members and the friends who support them. David said many of the fighters are blessed with people in their lives who love and care for them and are most likely concerned with what the future holds. By facing their condition with courage, determination, and perseverance, the fighters demonstrate life lessons that buoy everyone's spirits in the long run. Family members and friends also find support and encouragement from other spouses and caregivers with whom they have so much in common. The Rock Steady Boxing community is full of camaraderie and encouragement no matter how Parkinson's has affected one's life.

Because there was only one Rock Steady Boxing class at Reid Rehab initially, there was a wide range of ability among the fighters. One of the first people David met at the gym was a man named Craig who was a little older than David, and considerably less mobile. In fact, during that first session, Craig required a support person to help him get through the exercises. David said Craig was the nicest man anyone could hope to meet and that despite his limitations, Craig worked hard and eventually became a role model for everyone else in the gym.

Just before the closing huddle, when the fighters stand in a circle, hold hands, and shout, "Rock Steady!" David commended Craig on his effort and told him that he was an inspiration to work hard. "Craig's voice broke and tears came to his eyes. In fact, there wasn't a dry eye in the room," David recalled. "In a relatively short period of time, Craig could get up and down from the floor mat without needing the PT belt at all. The rest of us began to feel stronger and more hopeful as well. We came to see that we were more than just victims of our condition. We could help each other and help ourselves!"

Word of the Reid Rehab affiliate Rock Steady program spread, and more people came to see the program in action. Many of them stayed, and in no time at all, the coaches were able to add classes and divide the group into those who were more mobile and those who were less so. David said he worked out at the gym three times a week for 90 minutes per session and although he felt great and knew the exercises were good for him, they also wore him out. He was still working full time at the church and found it difficult to train at Rock Steady, rush home and shower, get something to eat, and then head back to the office without a break. Although he wanted to continue his ministry for as long as he could, he saw the writing on the wall. To continue focusing on his health, he needed to set aside a time to retire.

"Parkinson's definitely had an impact on that decision," David admitted. "I didn't want to be one of those poor souls I've known over the years. I want to maintain as much independence as possible, and Rock Steady Boxing is helping me do just that. My wife, Pam, is a wonderful support person who helps and encourages me, but I don't want to get to that point of total care yet. I'd rather that happen later as opposed to sooner."

David announced his retirement to his congregation and made plans with Pam to relocate to Noblesville, Indiana, where they could be near their two daughters and three grandchildren and David could work out at the Indianapolis Rock Steady Boxing headquarters. He told a newspaper reporter that he planned to watch sports and do some traveling; he also said that if his retirement was as blessed as his ministry, it was sure to be a wonderful new phase of life.

Naturally, the folks at First Presbyterian were sorry to see him go but came out in droves to say good-bye and wish him well when he conducted his final service on November 30, 2014. The congregation threw him a reception after the morning worship, and his friends at Rock Steady Boxing also gave the Laymans a farewell lunch. Although David would be missed at the gym, the others were excited that he would be able to continue his training in the place where it all began.

Today, David is a regular fixture around the Indianapolis Rock Steady gym, and even though he is convinced his technique is a challenge to the coaches, he's met a whole new group of friends, is in better shape than he was in his twenties, and, along with the combination of medications, has slowed the progress of his disease.

"If they ever made a video of how not to box, I would be the star of it," he laughed. "But I love Rock Steady Boxing and can see the difference it has made in my life. It's helping me get stronger every day, and that's good, because God isn't done with me yet."

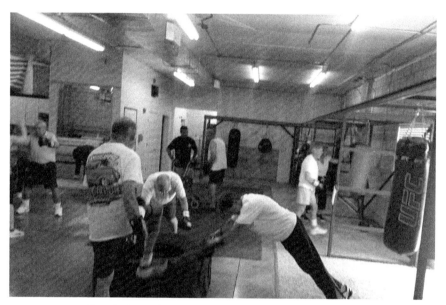

Rock Steady Boxing Carson City, Nevada

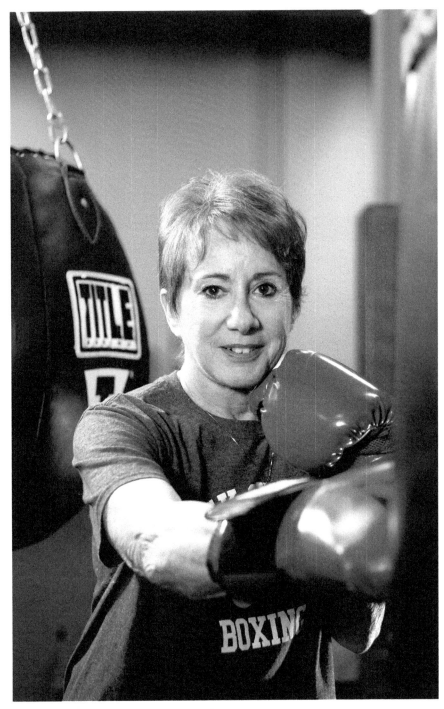

Linda Porter
Rock Steady Boxing Indianapolis

ROUND 8

Faith, Hope, and Love

"Even when things seemed so dim, I continued to push forward."
—Sugar Ray Leonard

The golden years of retirement were everything Linda Porter hoped they would be and more. After spending 25 years as a personnel recruiter, she was enjoying the fruits of her labor in an active adult lifestyle alongside her husband, Don. "We are not the kind of people to just sit around and watch TV now that we are not working full time. We were and continue to be very active people who enjoy a number of things, ranging from downhill skiing to jet skiing, waterskiing, rollerblading, dancing, and more."

Six years ago, the couple sold their home in sunny New Mexico and relocated to the quaint town of Zionsville, Indiana, where they could be near their two sons and enjoy their three beautiful granddaughters. The Porters found a gorgeous property on a golf course as well as a warm, wonderful church community that welcomed them with open arms. Life was practically perfect in every way until 2013, when

Linda began experiencing shoulder trouble and noticed a slight tremor in her hand.

Linda brought her symptoms to the attention of her doctor, who was treating her for an unrelated ankle injury. She assumed the strange phenomenon was a byproduct of her shoulder pain and wanted him to look at it after taking care of her ankle, but the physician disagreed. "I think you need to see another doctor," he told her.

"Oh no," she replied, dismissing his suggestion, "I'm sure it's all part of the same problem—"

The doctor wouldn't let her finish. He took her by the hand and looked her in the eye. "Linda, you have to see a neurologist," he stressed.

Linda remained skeptical, and when she returned home, she looked up "hand tremors" on the Internet, hoping to find a condition that would correlate to her shoulder pain. Everything she found seemed to point in one direction, however: Parkinson's disease.

Linda refused to believe that she could actually have Parkinson's. Although her experience with the condition was limited, those she had seen were unsmiling, frail beings who trembled involuntarily and were out of control where their bodies were concerned. Every once in a while, she would find articles related to benign tremors or pinched nerves, which convinced her that this was the most likely cause of her issues; when she finally saw a neurology specialist, she expected him to concur.

Unfortunately, he didn't. After conducting a routine exam, he told her the exact opposite. "I'm sorry to have to tell you this, but you have Parkinson's."

The 71-year-old sat in stunned silence, letting the word wash over her. She didn't know what to say or which questions to ask. She was still in a daze when she left the examination room and checked out at the reception desk a few minutes later. The receptionist noticed her pale complexion and asked if she was OK.

"No, I'm not," Linda stammered in reply. "The doctor just told me that I have Parkinson's disease."

The receptionist rose to her feet, came around the desk, and folded Linda into a hug. "I am so sorry," she told her. "I will keep you in my prayers."

Linda thanked the woman and numbly walked out to her car to call her husband, who was volunteering at their church that day. He had offered to clear his schedule and accompany his wife to her appointment, but because she had still believed it was nothing to be concerned about, she had told him a change in his schedule wasn't necessary. Now all she wanted was to hear his voice and feel his arms around her.

"What did the doctor say?" he asked when he answered the phone.

She took a breath and told him her diagnosis. "He said I have Parkinson's."

Don's response was immediate. "I'm on my way home," he promised.

The couple told their sons that same evening. Both sons gave their mother their unwavering love and support, but even with her family's strength surrounding her, Linda didn't feel like the same person anymore. She was a person with Parkinson's disease, and her condition consumed her.

She thought about it constantly. She developed every psychosomatic symptom imaginable. She worried that her life no longer had any value and wondered at what point her quality of life would diminish to the point that she was unrecognizable as the person she once had been.

"I was in a very dark place," she acknowledged. "On the outside, I tried to smile and have a positive attitude, but on the inside, I was sad and depressed. Everything I read about Parkinson's online scared me, and when I went to the doctor's office and saw other patients hobbling around on walkers and looked into their unsmiling faces, I wondered how long it would be before I joined their ranks."

Like other Parkinson's patients, Linda sought a second opinion to confirm her diagnosis. Her doctor started her on a regimen of medication to help with her initial symptoms and suggested exercise as a means to forestall those symptoms that had not occurred yet. Linda had no idea what type of exercise would be best, however. She turned once again to the Internet but found little help. Articles suggested brain games for mental acuity and dancing to help with balance, but she highly doubted crossword puzzles and Arthur Murray lessons would help her stay healthy in the long term.

She also eschewed the idea of joining a Parkinson's support group. She knew there was a lot of valuable information that could be shared in such a group and that some people found the groups to be very therapeutic, but she also knew it wasn't for her. "I had visions of a bunch of sick people sitting around talking about their problems, and I knew it would only make me feel worse," she said.

A little over a year after diagnosis, Linda's husband had knee-replacement surgery. While he was in the hospital,

Linda took the opportunity to visit a friend from church who happened to be an inpatient at the same location. In the course of conversation, Linda disclosed her condition, which prompted the other woman to tell her about a little boxing place she'd heard about that helped people with Parkinson's. She had another friend, Mary, who was also afflicted with the condition and was getting a lot out of the program. She gave Linda the woman's name and number and encouraged her to call. "When I did, we talked for over an hour," Linda said.

The "little boxing place" was Rock Steady Boxing, and after listening to Mary talk about the program, it didn't take long for Linda to check it out. At 4'11", Linda hardly fit the mold of a traditional prizefighter, but she knew that didn't matter. The program was designed for everyone, and she thought the whole thing sounded like a lot of fun. A few days later, she made the 30-minute drive to the Rock Steady Boxing headquarters in Indianapolis, walked into the lobby, and stopped dead in her tracks, unsure of what to do next.

"Rock Steady coach Christine Timberlake was the first person I met. She saw me standing there and asked how she could help me, and I just started crying," Linda said. "I told her, 'I have Parkinson's disease,' and she came right over and hugged me. I felt better right away."

Christine took Linda over to the Cornerman's Lounge, a comfortable visitors' area where guests can observe classes and see the Rock Steady Boxing program in action. Linda was in awe of the brightly painted gym, full-sized boxing ring, professional equipment, and diverse group of participants who seemed to be having the time of their lives. She couldn't wait to get started. She enrolled in the program and found everyone to be as upbeat as they had been on her first day there. They welcomed "Smurfette" as one of their own, and it didn't take long for Linda to start trading jabs (figuratively) with her fellow fighters.

Linda said Rock Steady proved to be more than a great exercise program. It was also the support group she needed to stay strong in her fight against Parkinson's. A lot of good-natured teasing and playful harassment goes on among the participants, as well as discussions about symptoms and disease progression. Linda says the camaraderie is beneficial for her mental health and enables her to talk to people who are going through the same thing from a position of empowerment rather than despair. "It's really effortless," she said.

Linda can already tell that she is getting stronger and healthier. No two workouts are exactly alike, and Linda never knows quite what to expect when she arrives for her class. Some days, the group may take baseball bats to old car tires, shoot baskets, or play volleyball. Other days may find the group performing calisthenics in a staff member's office as a joke. On still other days, they may begin their session by sharing personal stories or talking about life prior to Parkinson's. Linda says it's amazing what she learns about her fellow boxers. "I've been amazed at how many doctors, lawyers, ministers, and scientists were among us," she says. "Parkinson's really does affect a wide range of people."

Members of Rock Steady Boxing represent nearly every possible socioeconomic background, and across the spectrum, there are a diverse group of men and women whose lives have been changed by the disease and then changed once again by the discovery of Rock Steady Boxing, as well as the trainers who are committed to helping them with the fight. "You can tell that the trainers and coaches really love what they do," Linda said. "It's not just a job for them. Coaches Christine and Kristy really take the time to watch over us, help us get our technique down, and do the exercises right so that we can get the most from the workout and be better boxers. They also teach us how to take a fall, roll over, and get back up. It's very comprehensive. They really care about us, and it's wonderful."

Linda's family members are extremely supportive of their "champ" and have made the trek to the northeast-side facility to watch her in action. Don, her sons, and even her granddaughters can see how much she enjoys the program and the progress she has made since joining. Not only is she now able to do 37 push-ups, but she has also found her rhythm on the speed bag. In fact, she has become so proficient on the apparatus that Don bought her one for Valentine's Day so she can practice at home. It may not be the most romantic of gifts, but unlike roses that die in a week, her speed bag will stand the test of time.

Rock Steady Boxing has given Linda not only a way to combat her condition but also something to look forward to week after week. She said she cannot imagine there will ever be a time when she doesn't attend class, and she constantly champions the benefits of the program. She takes informational brochures to her physician's office, updates him on her condition, and does not hesitate to reach out to those who may need to know about the program.

During a recent reunion with several high school girl-friends, Linda noticed several familiar symptoms in one of them, and when the woman fainted in the bathroom, Linda told her she needed to go to the doctor. "I don't know what you are being treated for, but you have got to see a neurologist. If it turns out that you have Parkinson's, then you need to get to Rock Steady Boxing," she told her friend.

Linda says Rock Steady Boxing has changed her outlook on her diagnosis, and while there may not be a cure for Parkinson's, the program helps her feel better about her prognosis. She has met the most wonderful people, has lessened the symptoms she was experiencing, and has become more optimistic and hopeful about what the future holds. "I was lucky because I was diagnosed later in life," she said. "I was originally told that I maybe had 10 years of quality life left, but now I am told I will probably live to be 100. That's nice to hear, but I really don't fear it at all. I don't give Parkinson's that kind of power over me anymore."

The staff at Rock Steady Boxing found Linda's story so inspirational that they asked her to speak at the organization's annual fundraiser. Although she was nervous, she agreed to tell the 700 people assembled about the difference Rock Steady Boxing has made in her life. As Linda addressed the crowd, she said, "I literally walked out of the dark and into the sunshine. ... I could feel the hope take over my mind. That day, *my* light was turned back on. ... Of course no one would ever choose to have Parkinson's disease, but along with the bad, there has been a lot of good. (At Rock steady Boxing) the good comes from the coaches, the staff, and the boxers. We are all in this fight together. If I had not developed Parkinson's, I would have missed getting to know these incredibly amazing people, and that would have been a terrible loss. Life is funny that way ... it takes away and then it gives something back."

Linda believes that God does not give you more than you can handle and that when life throws you to the ground, you can't give up, you have to fight the fight. If she had not moved to Indiana, she would not have joined her church community and may never have met the person who would tell her about Rock Steady Boxing, so she truly feels the move was all part of God's plan for her life. Thanks to Rock Steady Boxing, she says, she is no longer trembling, is more agile, and is in the best shape she can be in. "I have met a great group of people who I can laugh with, and I am no longer depressed. Rock Steady Boxing is the rock that I cling to. It gives me hope, and if you don't have hope, you have nothing."

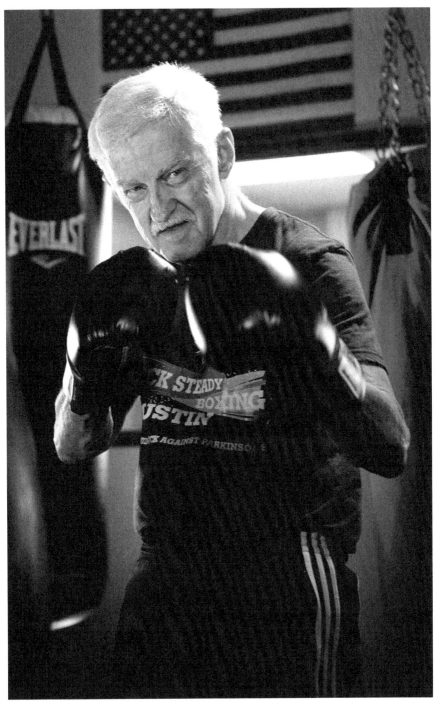

Rodger Dalston
Rock Steady Boxing Austin

The Best Medicine

"I don't want to be no more than what I am."

—Joe Frazier

If that which does not kill us makes us stronger, then Dr. Rodger Millard Dalston should be indestructible by now. In fact, by the time he was diagnosed with Parkinson's disease in 2000, the former university professor had been handed enough hard knocks to cause even the toughest prizefighter to tap out. But thanks to a positive attitude, a wicked sense of humor, and the comedic timing of Milton Berle, Rodger refuses to wallow in self-pity. "Life is too important to be taken seriously," he said.

Born to parents Beatrice and Millard Dalston of Maplewood, New Jersey, Rodger came into the world with a deformed right leg that was significantly shorter than his left. He endured seven surgeries within the first three years of his life in hopes of correcting the limb deformity and tried to learn to walk by using a special shoe designed to compensate for the short leg. When he continued to struggle, however, his doctor talked to his parents about having the leg amputated.

"They initially resisted, arguing that they would prefer to wait until I was a teenager and could decide for myself if I wanted to keep the leg or lose it," Rodger said. "Fortunately, the physician's argument won out. He correctly surmised that if I waited, I would consider the leg an integral part of me and would never have it amputated, even if it would brand me as a deformed person in both body and spirit."

At the age of four and a half, the troublesome leg was removed and Rodger adjusted to life with a prosthetic limb. The new hardware wasn't always easy to maneuver, but it did not prevent him from participating in youth sports or other activities. Rodger said his parents raised him in a loving and supportive environment that left him with the impression that even if he couldn't do something that other kids could do, he certainly had the right to try. As a result, he earned the swimmer's rank of shark at the local YMCA, participated fully in gym class from kindergarten forward, played intramural basketball throughout high school, and was a member of the Maplewood lacrosse team for one year.

Rodger loved lacrosse and was looking forward to another great season on the field, but something happened that second year that changed his lacrosse career forever. In one of the most heartbreaking experiences of his life, Rodger arrived for practice and was told he could no longer participate. The explanation was short, to the point, and brutally honest: members of the US Navy B team refused to play against Maplewood if Rodger was on the team.

"After almost 60 years, I still remember the tears that welled up in my eyes as I walked back to my beloved two-tone '53 Ford," he recalled. "I sat behind the wheel and cried for about five minutes. After that, I wiped the tears from my eyes, looked toward the lacrosse practice field, said, 'To heck with you all,' and drove home. Naturally, the words I really used were a little more graphic, but those are best not repeated."

If that weren't enough to justify a lifetime membership into the Woe Is Me Program (WIMP), Rodger has also endured two operations to open blocked cardiac arteries, undergone a right lung lobectomy to remove a cancerous tumor, experienced the pain of suture removal following bilateral blepharoplasty so he could see well enough to drive again, and had a hernia repair so he could get back in the gym and perform exercises that would help him maintain his core and keep his balance. In addition, he suffers from obstructive sleep apnea. Despite all of the maladies, Rodger has never let his tough luck get him down. "I make a concerted effort to maintain a positive attitude toward life. It's not a façade. I love to laugh, and I love to make others laugh, but don't misunderstand; I'm not a mindless idiot, even if my wife thinks I am on occasion," he said.

His wife is Eileen, a woman he met when they both entered the graduate Communication Sciences and Disorders program at Northwestern University. It took Rodger about "five nanoseconds" to fall in love with her, but it took Eileen nearly 10 months to reciprocate his feelings. She initially saw Rodger as a good friend who could make her laugh. After nearly 49 years of marriage, it's clear they remain the best of friends. Rodger said that he still makes his wife laugh like no one else can and the couple can be pretty silly when they are home alone. "In fact, we are certain that if we ever move into a retirement facility, they will have to lock us up in separate padded apartments."

Throughout his adult life, Rodger kept up a steady stream of activity. During their tenure in Chapel Hill, he and Eileen have spent many wonderful days in North Carolina and in Georgia running the rapids in an outrigger canoe. He learned to snow ski on one leg, an activity he continued even after his Parkinson's diagnosis. In fact, he periodically threatened to wear a t-shirt over his winter jacket that would alert other skiers that he had missing brain tissues as well as a missing leg. "It would read, 'This is nothing, I also have Parkinson's,'" he said.

Rodger's journey with Parkinson's began with a telltale tremor in the spring of 1999. Because of his background in language pathology, he had a working knowledge of Parkinson's as it pertained to speech anomalies and was certain of his diagnosis; however, in 2000, he decided to seek a second opinion. Rodger visited the world-renowned Dr. Joseph Jankovic at the Parkinson's Disease Center and Movement Disorders Clinic at the Baylor College of Medicine in Houston, Texas, and with Eileen sitting beside him, he began the tests necessary for a full evaluation. During the consultation, Dr. Jankovic asked Rodger to extend both arms and spread his fingers as wide as possible. Rodger knew what the doctor was looking for and prepared his wife for the inevitable. Sure enough, when he did what the specialist asked, his arm began to flutter wildly.

"Well, if the air conditioner breaks down, I'll still have a fan to keep me cool," Eileen commented wryly.

A few minutes later, Dr. Jankovic attempted to test Rodger for cogwheel rigidity in his right leg, the one that had been amputated several decades before. As the doctor reached for the limb, Rodger joked that if he found cogwheel rigidity in that particular leg, he would stop by a service station on the way home and get a lube job.

The neurologist turned to the couple and chuckled. "Well, at least you both have a sense of humor," he said.

For Rodger, having a sense of humor is more than simply being able to laugh in the face of adversity; it is his lifeline. Although his physician may be able to prescribe any number of pharmaceuticals to help alleviate the symptoms of Parkinson's disease, Rodger knows that his quips and one-liners are the things that help him get through the day-to-day grind. For Rodger, laughter is truly the best medicine, and he constantly looks for the light side of every adversity.

"If you want to know a secret, I actually think Eileen and our son, Scott, are responsible for my condition," Rodger joked. "Eileen wrote her master's thesis on Parkinson's disease and its impact on speech, and our son, wishing to improve his chances of entering medical school, worked in a lab that was analyzing Parkinson's data. There may be a few flaws in this theory, of course, but that's my story and I'm sticking to it."

After the formal diagnosis, Rodger continued to teach at the University of Texas at Austin. His symptoms were such that the disease did not significantly impair his interaction in the classroom and clinic setting, though on occasion, it did make itself known. He recalled a class during which he picked up a bottle of water and his hand shook so vigorously that water splashed out of the container and hit a couple of students. Rodger apologized for the accident, shrugged, and then proceeded to walk around the room "anointing" the rest of the students as well.

While teaching a course on research design, Rodger had a moment in which he divulged his condition in answer to a student's question about p-values, or rejection levels, in a research project. He said he never had a more attentive class than he did when he cited a Parkinson's drug study and how he would evaluate the rejection levels as both a patient and a researcher. He said the discussion ran well beyond the class hour as the students talked about a variety of topics, including benefit/risk management, power analysis, and more. "Even though that class was held over 13 years ago, I would venture to guess that many of them retain a good deal of the information that was covered because it was so personalized," he said. "The class probably would have been a bust if I did not have the disease, so let's hear it for Parkinson's. On occasion, it comes in handy."

Rodger retired in 2004, and although he tried to maintain a consistent routine of physical exercise, he stayed home more often than he went to the gym. He knew that vigorous exercise would lead to a rush of endorphins and help him feel better, but finding the motivation to do it was a challenge. As a result, his condition progressed. He said he knew he had to do something when he received a call from *Sesame Street* asking him to be the poster child for the lowercase *r* because of the way he slouched and tilted forward. "My posture was so bad, especially in the car, that I could not be seen," Rodger said. "People frequently rolled down their windows and asked if my parents knew their six-year-old was driving a vehicle."

In the fall of 2015, Rock Steady Boxing was featured on CBS's *Sunday Morning* with Leslie Stahl. A friend of Rodger's saw the segment and told him about this exciting "new" program to combat Parkinson's disease that was limited to eight gyms throughout the country. Rodger assumed that with his luck, the nearest gym would be 2,500 miles away but was pleased to discover there was a Rock Steady facility in Austin and only seven miles from his home.

"I had plenty of boxing experience as a child, because my parents provided me with a punching bag in the form of my sister Gayle, who was six years older than I," he joked. "In classic sibling-rivalry form, we sparred constantly. She thought she should have the last word in any argument because she was the oldest, and I knew I should have it because I was male. It's a wonder she didn't hate me while we were growing up."

Rodger drove over to the Rock Steady Boxing Austin gym and fell in love with the program, the class, and the instructor right away. Unlike other exercise classes in which the biggest challenge is to rotate one's head through a range of 90 degrees, Rock Steady Boxing coach Kristi Richards encourages her clients to push themselves. She does it in such a way that no one is embarrassed by his or her limitations. In addition, Kristi cultivates a very warm environment where everyone feels like family.

After that first class, Rodger was completely wiped out. In fact, he said he felt as though he had been put through an old-fashioned wringer. Although the rigor of the classes have not diminished in any way, he says he is in better physical shape than he was at the beginning and can withstand the workouts without getting as tired.

"What distinguishes the Rock Steady Boxing classes from other forms of exercise is the fact that I actually look forward to them," he said. "The exercise rigor and the camaraderie are such that the only classes I have missed have been ones that conflict with previously scheduled appointments."

Kristi Richards, owner of Rock Steady Boxing Austin, said that from the moment she met Rodger, she was struck by his intelligence, wit, and dedication to excellence. No matter what she asks of the class, she can count on Rodger to be the first fighter to attempt it. He often stays after class to practice jumping rope, and he is determined not to let Parkinson's disease get the best of him. "Rodger is an over-achiever in every good sense of the word," she said. "He doesn't quit, and he brings such a charm to the class that he is one of our most beloved fighters. He has come so far in his abilities, and I see him getting better day by day. He stands taller. His balance has improved, and he just doesn't quit."

Though he has been with Rock Steady Boxing for only a short time, Rodger feels good about his participation. He says Parkinson's is merely another trial in a lifetime of tests. With Rock Steady Boxing, he is ready to confront those challenges head on.

"I suppose this early in the game, it would be foolhardy of me to suggest that my symptoms have disappeared and that I am ready to get back out on the slopes," he said. "Of course, come to think of it, at 73 years of age, I'm on a slip-pery slope already that has nothing to do with Parkinson's. Whether my improvements are large or small at this point, I feel better about myself. If I can keep doing what I am doing and keep laughing, I will continue to be a happy man."

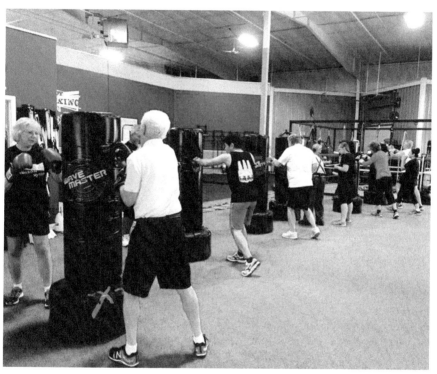

Rock Steady Boxing Madison, Wisconsin

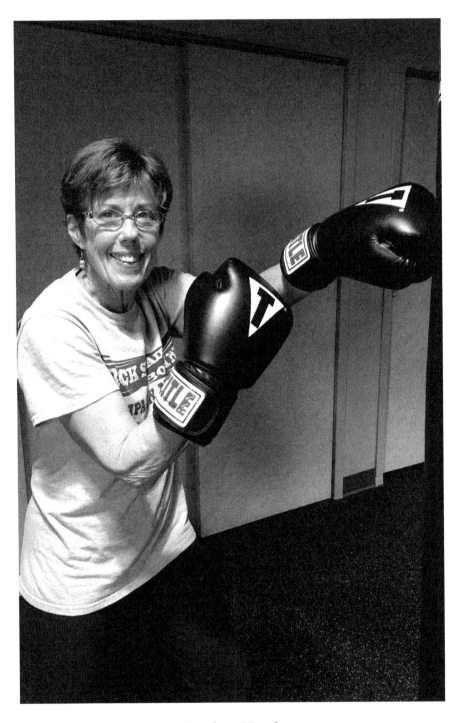

Lindsay Hood
Rock Steady Boxing Tampa Bay Area

ROUND 10

On My Own Two Feet

"When I am boxing ... I feel mentally and physically strong."
—Liam Hemsworth

Nurses are truly the unsung heroes of the healthcare profession. Every day, all over the world, they perform myriad tasks in a wide variety of settings with one goal in mind: to improve the lives of the people they serve. Not only do they save lives, bring healing to the infirmed, advocate for patients' rights, and help people die with dignity, but they are often the first to step up in times of crisis or to fulfill a role wherever there is a need.

That is the kind of nurse Lindsay Hood of Clearwater, Florida, wanted to be, and before her retirement in 2003, that's exactly the kind of nurse she was. Not only did she hold positions in a wide range of clinical settings and private practice, but she also followed her vocation to the halls of academia, where she did a stint as a nurse for a local high school.

Being a school nurse is never easy, and Lindsay quickly learned that she dispensed as much practical advice as medication and healed broken hearts along with bumps and bruises. "I really miss those kids sometimes," she said. "The more I worked around them, the more I wanted to know about them, and eventually, I went back to school to get my master's degree so that I could become a guidance counselor."

Even after she left the workforce, Lindsay continued to be active. She was at the gym two days a week, where she did Pilates, did yoga, and swam. She spent time with John, a retired orthopedist, as well as her two grown sons, and she also cycled, went horseback riding, and created a network of friends with whom she could have lunch, shop, and socialize. "I was pretty lucky to be able to do all of those things," she said.

By November 2005, however, Lindsay had noticed a change in her overall health. She felt tired, whereas she used to feel full of energy. She shuffled when she walked and had trouble keeping her balance. She experienced some cognitive issues as well as some memory lapses. Her left arm rose of its own accord and had to be manually lowered. After falling a few times, Lindsay decided to see a doctor to find out what was wrong. "My husband didn't really notice anything out of the ordinary, but I'd been in the healthcare profession long enough to know that I needed to follow up on these symptoms and not let them get any worse," she said.

Lindsay consulted with Dr. Michael Andriola, a movement disorder specialist and board-certified neurologist in Clearwater who had experience in a number of conditions including Parkinson's disease. Dr. Andriola had Lindsay walk up and down the hallway in his office in order to evaluate her gait, and then he suggested a round of the antiparkinson drug Mirapex in hopes that it would make a difference.

Lindsay took the medication and said it helped. She felt better, saw some significant improvements in her symptoms, and wasn't as tired as she had been in recent months. "That's how it was determined that I had Parkinson's disease," she said. "I reacted positively to the medication."

Although she had a background in the clinical field, Lindsay said she didn't know much about Parkinson's disease. In light of her diagnosis, however, she was eager to learn more. She scoured the Internet for additional information and the latest research on the subject and discovered that exercise was critical to preventing disease progression. Lindsay was thrilled to keep up with her regular workouts when she could, took her medication religiously, and checked in with her doctor as recommended.

Everything seemed fine, but looking back on the early days after her diagnosis, Lindsay admitted that she was in a state of denial at the time. As someone dealing with a life-altering condition, she went through a range of thoughts and feelings about her situation but sought no help from others. She saw no purpose in surrounding herself with other Parkinson's patients, listening to their problems or envisioning an uncertain future. It was as if she could avoid the disease itself by avoiding others with it, not realizing how invaluable that camaraderie and support could be. "I now know that you can learn a lot from others who have the disease," she said. "In fact, one of the best ways to learn about Parkinson's disease is to be around others who have it."

If Lindsay was in a state of denial, then her family was not faring any better. John and the twins had always been the kind of men who kept their cards close to the chest, but after a while, their keep-calm-and-carry-on attitude led to hurt feelings and plenty of frustration. Lindsay wanted to talk about her condition, but she didn't know how to broach the subject when her husband and sons were too busy acting as if nothing had changed. After months of keeping her feelings bottled up inside, she finally began to share more about her situation. "I didn't want them to treat me any differently or to do things that I could obviously do for myself, but I needed them to understand what I was going through so that they could help me when necessary or just listen if I needed to talk."

For several years, Lindsay's medications and regular workouts were enough to keep her Parkinson's symptoms from progressing too rapidly, but by 2015, those efforts plateaued. Her doctor adjusted her medications to a time-release formula, but she knew she needed to find a new kind of workout to give her brain a boost.

Luckily for Lindsay, her massage therapist had heard about Rock Steady Boxing Tampa Bay Area and encouraged her to give it a try.

Lindsay wasn't sure what to think. She had always thought of boxing as dangerous and violent and had never been a fan of the sport. Still, she was intrigued enough to drive over to the gym owned by Tara Schwartz and located in the Bodyssey Performance/Advanced Physical Therapy Center in Largo, Florida, to check it out. After all, nothing else was working for her at the time; perhaps the Rock Steady Boxing program would make a difference.

"The first time I walked into the gym, I thought, *My gosh, we are all such different ages. How could we all be helped by the same boxing program?* she said.

As she took part in that initial class, Lindsay realized it had been a while since she had been around such an energetic and enthusiastic group of people. Everything about the Rock Steady Boxing program in Tampa Bay was upbeat and high-energy. The boxers were enthusiastically fighting back against Parkinson's, and the coaches were dedicated to helping them as much as possible. "I knew something good was going on here, and I was excited to be part of it." Schwartz said Lindsay's reaction was typical of what happens to someone when they see the Rock Steady Boxing program for the first time: They may not know what to expect when they walk in, but they can't forget what they've seen once they leave.

As a personal trainer for more than two decades, Schwartz had read up on studies that showed a correlation between vigorous exercise and its effect on Parkinson's symptoms, and she wanted to learn more. After hearing about Rock Steady Boxing, Schwartz had traveled to Indianapolis to see the program for herself, and what she saw impressed her. "I hadn't been that amazed … in my life," she said. "It was just one of the most amazing things I've ever been a part of. I probably saw 120 boxers there over a three-day period, and I was just in awe. I just knew that once I saw it being done there, that I had to bring it back here."

Schwartz opened her affiliate program in October 2015, and it didn't take long for boxers to find out about it. She says she typically has 12–15 participants in each Rock Steady Boxing class and when they are in the gym, their condition is the last thing on participants' minds. "They are empowered. There is no medicine that can give that kind of hope to people. And if I can be a facilitator of that, then that's what I feel like I need to do," she said.

Dr. Andriola was all in favor of Lindsay joining Rock Steady Boxing Tampa Bay Area. He knew how much exercise had helped her in the past and was confident that this new routine would give her the added benefit she needed to put her Parkinson's symptoms on the back burner. Her family also got behind the new fitness program and gave her their full support.

"The guys still aren't very forthcoming with their emotions, but they are guys, and deep down inside, I know they get a kick out of it," Lindsay said. "Come to find out, one of my sons actually learned some boxing when he was a young man, so he thought it was cool that I was becoming a puncher as well." Lindsay said that in addition to being designed for people with Parkinson's disease, the workout offers boxers a positive experience that serves the body, mind, and spirit. She said a certain confidence comes over her when she puts on her gloves, gets into the boxer stance, and hits the heavy bag with all of her might. Not only does she "feel cool" with every jab, cross, and hook, but it is then that she is able to feel in control of an uncontrollable situation.

"It feels good and it really brings you out of your shell," she said. "I didn't realize how angry I was until I started hitting the bag, but deep down, there was a part of me that wondered why this happened to me. What did I do to deserve this? And what could I have done differently? I didn't let any of that out until I lit into that bag, let the tears flow, and allowed the emotions to take over. Rock Steady Boxing is not only good for you physically, but it's therapeutic as well. It does a lot for your mental and emotional well-being."

But the exercises are only part of the equation. Lindsay said ever since she joined Rock Steady Boxing Tampa Bay Area, she has met a number of kind and wonderful people who have helped her become a champion in her fight. Not only does she credit Schwartz for bringing Rock Steady Boxing to the area, but she also says Coach Jordan Whittemore has been instrumental in helping her succeed in the program. "[Jordan] is just fabulous. Like all of the coaches, she knew a lot and helped me feel good about myself right away. She knows how to give me the encouragement I need, and when I walk out of here, I feel great," Lindsay said. "Once upon a time, the future looked shaky, but I know I can get better by following this program. Thanks to Rock Steady Boxing, I am taking care of myself and standing on my own two feet."

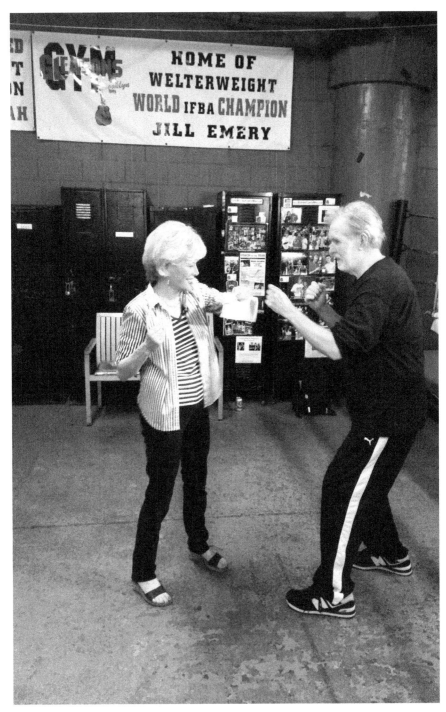

Lesley Stahl and Aaron Latham
Rock Steady Boxing NY/LA

The Knockout Punch

"To be a champion you have to believe in yourself when no one else does."
—Sugar Ray Robinson

When Aaron Latham was growing up in the tiny town of Spur, Texas, boxing was a big part of his life. He not only listened to the Friday-night fights on the radio and accompanied his father to the local Golden Glove matches but also had a ring set up in his home and used to invite his pals over for friendly bouts. He said he used to dream of the day when he could execute the moves of his favorite boxer, Sugar Ray Robinson. "My greatest ambition was to knock someone out, but at the age of 10, 11, and 12, I didn't have the muscle mass to pull it off," he said.

By the time Aaron was in high school, his fascination with boxing had waned and he turned his attention to the football field. His father was a high school football coach, and Aaron dreamed of gridiron greatness, but a destroyed kidney sidelined his prep-school football career.

Luckily, Aaron was a good student who excelled in all of his classes; he was ultimately accepted to Amherst College in

Massachusetts. He did well at the private liberal arts school, where he fell in love with journalism, became the editor of *The Student* newspaper, and earned his undergraduate degree in 1966. He went on to do his graduate work at Princeton and, while completing his doctorate in English literature, took a summer internship at the *Washington Post*. Upon his graduation, the internship became a full-time position.

"I sat at a desk right beside Carl Bernstein," Aaron recalled. "When I left the *Post* to take a position at *Esquire* in New York, another guy moved into my old desk. His name was Bob Woodward."

After a stint at *Esquire*, Aaron moved on to *New York* magazine, where, in 1973, he was asked to do a column on the Watergate scandal. He traveled to Washington on a Saturday, but everyone was out of town for the weekend. Desperate for some anecdotal information to help with his story, he reached out to a former *Washington Post* colleague who suggested he contact Lesley Stahl, then a rookie reporter for CBS. Aaron called Lesley on Sunday night at home and told her of his dilemma, but she had no pity on her fellow journalist. "She said, 'If this is really about work, call me at the office,' and slammed the phone down," he recalled. "I promised myself I would never speak to her again in my whole life, but the next day, I was getting nowhere with my reporting, so I called her again—this time at the office. I told her who I was and what I was up to, and she said, 'Oh. ... Want to have dinner?'"

The two made arrangements to meet the following evening, and in an effort to put a face with the name, Aaron turned on the TV to see what Lesley looked like. "She was so beautiful. My heart stopped, my mouth dried up, and I said, 'What have I gotten myself into?'" he recalled in a 1977 interview with *People* magazine.

The two saw each other socially over the next two years. He traveled from New York to Washington to cover the events leading to Nixon's resignation, but he and Lesley weren't officially dating. Finally, when they no longer had the Watergate scandal holding them together, they realized there was more below the surface. "Suddenly we started seeing something different from what we had been seeing—almost like the old story of the boss who married his secretary after 35 years," Lesley told *People* in 1977.

Aaron moved into Lesley's apartment on Christmas of 1976, and the following February, they had a low-key wedding. Soon after, the newlyweds also became the parents of a beautiful baby girl, Taylor Stahl Latham. The two journalists initially lived in Georgetown, and Aaron returned to *Esquire*, spending a few days a month writing in the New York editorial offices.

In 1978, he wrote an article called "The Ballad of the Urban Cowboy," the story of a strange love triangle between a boy, a girl, and a mechanical bull. Set in a large Houston honky-tonk, it's a unique look at the breakdown of love when the girl turns out to be a better bull rider than the guy. Not long after the story was published, Hollywood came calling. Aaron struck a deal that would enable him to cowrite the screenplay for the film that would eventually star John Travolta and Debra Winger.

Urban Cowboy came out in 1980 and received generally positive reviews from the critics. The film helped country music reach a crossover audience and was nominated for two

Golden Globe Awards, a BAFTA Award, and a Grammy for best motion picture soundtrack album. After the success of *Urban Cowboy*, Aaron's star continued to rise. He left *Esquire* for a stint at *Rolling Stone*, where he penned profiles on a variety of luminaries including Warren Beatty, Paul Newman, and Elizabeth Taylor.

In 1983, he wrote a piece titled "Looking for Mr. Goodbody" about the rise of health clubs as the new singles scene of the '80s. Given the fitness craze that had captivated the decade, it is no surprise that Hollywood saw the potential in the story and was eager to cash in. Columbia Pictures bought the rights to the piece and commissioned Aaron to compose the screenplay. The plot line was centered somewhat on the story behind the story: A young writer goes undercover to dive into the sex-charged atmosphere of L.A.'s Sports Connection gym and pens a typical exposé but unwittingly falls in love with the gym's aerobics instructor, and when he decides to change the angle of the story, his editors do a rewrite, which infuriates him. The movie was called *Perfect* and also starred John Travolta in the leading role. Jamie Lee Curtis portrayed his love interest.

Like *Urban Cowboy*, *Perfect* received relatively positive reviews from the critics, but it was not as successful as some of Travolta's other movies. Still, Aaron was making a name for himself as a screenwriter, and it wasn't long before he was tapped for his next big project. "After I finished *Perfect*, Sam Goldwyn asked me if I wanted to write a screenplay about college football," Aaron said.

Being a Texas native as well as the son of a football coach, Aaron jumped at the chance to take a year off and travel the country to research various athletic departments at colleges and universities. He learned a lot, which resulted in the 1993 movie *The Program*, starring James Caan and Halle Berry. The film's story line centers on the fictional ESU Timberwolves and their quest for a bowl berth at any cost. The movie grossed $23 million in the United States, and although the reviews were mixed, it attracted a lot of fans, including critic Roger Ebert, who gave the film three out of four stars.

Aaron was not only busy with his journalism and screen-writing endeavors but had also become an author, penning such works as *The Frozen Leopard: Hunting My Dark Heart in Africa* (1991), *The Ballad of Gussie & Clyde* (1997), *The Code of the West* (2001), *The Cowboy with the Tiffany Gun* (2005), and *Riding with John Wayne* (2008). He was still very active, as well, but he began to feel a little awkward and was having a hard time putting on his coat. He mentioned the problem to his physician, but the doctor didn't seem overly concerned about it.

As time went on, Aaron's situation only got worse. "I started walking slower than I used to," he said. "My wife was always yelling at me to keep up, and for a while, I thought she was walking faster, but as it turned out, the problem was me."

Aaron returned to his doctor and was put through a battery of tests to evaluate his movements and check for neuro-sensitivity and reactions. He was asked to rise from a chair and to walk up and down the hallway on his heels so the doctor could check his gait. He was diagnosed with Parkinson's in 2009.

Aaron said he really knew nothing about Parkinson's when his doctor gave him the news, but he said the diagnosis wasn't presented as though it were the end of the world. He was told that the symptoms could be treated but the disease itself had no cure. Aaron said he was under the impression that Parkinson's was something that he had to pay attention to and to work on but that if he had known anything beyond that, he might have felt as though he had fallen off a cliff or something. "I was protected by my own ignorance," he laughed.

Although Aaron's symptoms were relatively mild, his doctor started him on antiparkinson medication. The doctor also suggested exercise to help keep Aaron's Parkinson's symptoms at bay, so Aaron spent time lifting weights and working out on the treadmill, but he found the routine monotonous, tiresome, and not as effective as he had hoped.

In early 2015, Aaron's son-in-law told him about a story he had heard on NPR about a boxing program that was good for people with Parkinson's disease. Aaron took down the information, and Lesley wasted no time in getting on the computer to find out more. She learned that the program was called Rock Steady Boxing, had been developed in Indianapolis, and could be found in a number of gyms throughout the world. By now, the couple was living in New York, and the only affiliate in the Big Apple was at the famed Gleason's Gym in Brooklyn.

Owned by Bruce Silverglade, Gleason's Gym is the oldest active boxing gym in the country. It opened in 1937 and enjoys a storied history. It is the gym where Muhammad Ali (then Cassius Clay) trained for his first fight against Sonny Liston in 1964 and that champions such as Mike Tyson and

Michael Spinks have called home over the years. In addition, Gleason's has served as the backdrop for movies such as *Raging Bull*, starring Robert De Niro, and *Million Dollar Baby*, starring Clint Eastwood. "It's a great old gym," Aaron said. "There are five rings and a diverse group of people doing extraordinary exercises in there. It's quite a scene."

Three times a week, Gleason's donated one of its rings to the Rock Steady Boxing NY/LA affiliate, which was run by the husband-and-wife team of Roberta Marongiu and Alex Montaldo. Marongiu is a researcher at Weill Cornell Medical College in New York who had been working on gene therapies for Parkinson's but was eager to do something to help people with Parkinson's in the present. She first heard about Rock Steady Boxing at a medical conference, thought it was a brilliant idea, and could not wait to get involved. She and Montaldo, who is an actor, traveled to Indianapolis to become certified Rock Steady Boxing coaches.

"She is a slave driver," Aaron said of Marongiu.

Aaron began working out at Rock Steady Boxing NY/LA in February 2015, and it wasn't long before he saw some significant improvement in his Parkinson's symptoms. He shook less. He moved more easily and felt a little better. Lesley also saw a change and went down to the gym to watch Aaron train. When she saw the Rock Steady Boxing program in action, she knew it would make a great story.

"I could not believe how arduous the hour is," Lesley told Marongiu.

Lesley returned with a CBS News film crew to interview the boxers and coaches and to capture footage of the Rock Steady Boxing method. She also interviewed with

Stephanie Combs-Miller, Director of Research, Krannert School of Physical Therapy, University of Indianapolis, who conducted the first study of how boxing therapy affects Parkinson 's disease, to learn why Dr. Combs-Miller thinks it works.

"We studied people over a two-year period who participated in boxing, and we didn't see any progression of the disease in the people that boxed," Dr. Combs-Miller said. "In fact, in some cases they were better … it enhances the uptake of the dopamine in the brain. It can improve growth of neurons."

Lesley's *CBS Sunday Morning* segment about Rock Steady Boxing aired on November 8, 2015. It had a tremendous impact on enrollment at Rock Steady Boxing affiliates throughout the country. Aaron said that prior to the segment airing, Rock Steady Boxing NY/LA had been a struggling program with only five fighters but in the months since the story aired, it has grown to 70 fighters. Lesley's CBS segment has been nominated for an Emmy.

"It seemed like everyone saw that piece," Aaron said. "Even neighbors I'd never met saw me out walking my dog and said, 'Weren't you on television the other day?'"

In the time that he has been with the Rock Steady Boxing program, Aaron said the folks at the gym have become like a second family to him and he has grown especially close to Marongiu and Montaldo. He said the changes he has seen in the people around the gym have been nothing short of incredible. Aaron says it is cathartic to literally fight back against Parkinson's disease, exciting to revisit the sport he loved as a child, and therapeutic to be around others like him who are fighting back for camaraderie and support.

"Rock Steady Boxing perks you up. It gives you a better attitude, and it's good for you," he said. "Parkinson's is the kind of condition that tries to make you smaller, but at Rock Steady Boxing, you can feel big again."

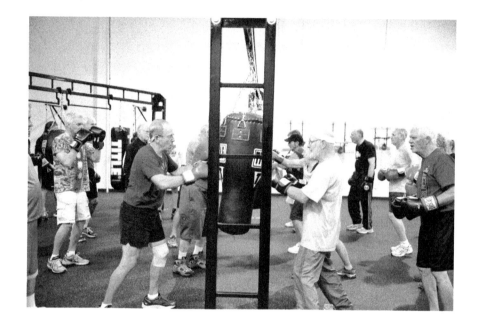

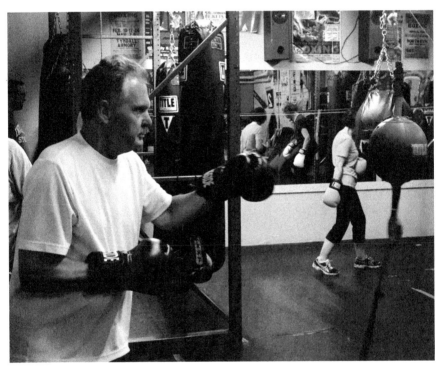

Rock Steady Boxing Terre Haute, Indiana

ACKNOWLEDGMENTS

Julie Young

First and foremost, I thank Joyce Johnson, Rock Steady Boxing Executive Director, for contacting me about this project and then commissioning me to write it. I connected with you immediately, was inspired by what I witnessed, and knew I would have a lot of fun telling the story of Rock Steady Boxing and the various people affected by this incredible program. You have been a dream to work with.

I also thank the men and women affiliated with the Rock Steady Boxing organization who gave me the profound privilege of telling their stories. I know it is difficult to entrust a complete stranger with your raw and innermost feelings. I hope you know how seriously I took my role in this project. You have all inspired me in ways you cannot imagine, and I am rooting for each and every one of you!

Thanks also to my editors and clients who were thrilled to learn that I had been given the opportunity to write this book and bent over backward to ensure that my workload remained bearable over these past few months. They include Sarah, Jodi, Vicki, Sue, Lauren, Dave, and Laura. I promise, I will be back to the grind very soon. You guys are the best!

Last but not least, I thank the three men in my life who are always in my corner, who give me a pep talk when I need it, give me tough love even when I don't want it, and listen to me talk endlessly about whatever project I happen to be working on: my husband, Shawn, and our sons, Chris and Vincent. They take over the daily responsibilities when I am overwhelmed, keep me laughing even when I feel like crying, and never count me out of the fight. You are the reason I continue to "go for it."

Marc Morrison

Rock Steady Boxing thanks photographer Marc Morrison for sharing his incredible talent as a volunteer photographer for the individual photos in this publication. On Sunday morning, November 8, 2015, CBS aired its cover story, "Fighting Back Against Parkinson's—in the ring," featuring Lesley Stahl in an interview with her husband, a Rock Steady boxer. Marc was emotionally touched by the story and wanted to do something to help. He called Rock Steady's headquarters and learned about this book. Marc has since traveled around the country, photographing the men and women profiled in *I Am Rock Steady.* We couldn't be more grateful for the skill with which he has captured their spirit and courage in his beautiful pictures. Thank you, Marc. (To view more of Marc's work, visit www.marcmorrison.com)

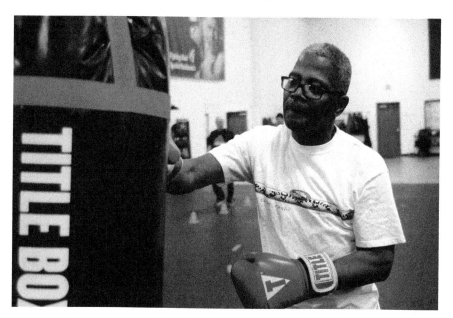

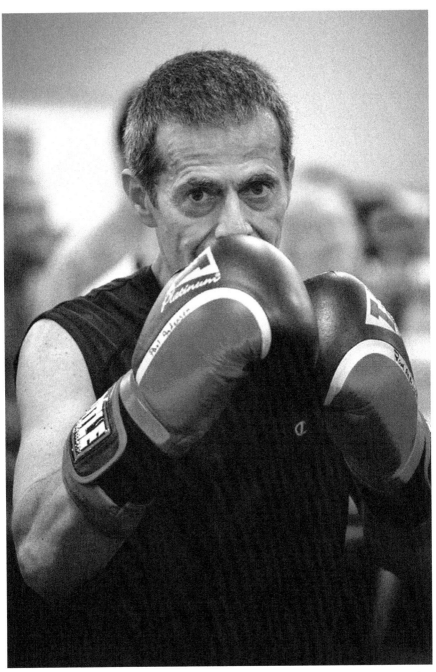

Photo by Lisa Boncosky

Rock Steady Boxing

Fighting Back Against Parkinson's Disease

Rock Steady Boxing, a 501(c)3 nonprofit organization founded in Indianapolis in 2006, gives hope to people with Parkinson's disease by improving their quality of life through a noncontact, boxing-inspired fitness curriculum.

In 2006, former Marion County Prosecutor Scott Newman was diagnosed with Parkinson's disease. He experienced a rapid progression of symptoms, including tremors, rigidity, and a loss of some functions. A friend taught him to box, and he quickly saw his symptoms decrease. After only a few weeks, he stretched out his arms and said, "Look, I'm Rock Steady," and Rock Steady Boxing was born.

In the United States, 1.5 million people have been diagnosed with Parkinson's and 60,000 more are diagnosed each year. National Parkinson's organizations have invested hundreds of millions of dollars in research to find a cause and a cure, but to date, they've been unsuccessful. It may be years before a cure is found, and decades more before a treatment is approved—but people with Parkinson's need help *today*.

Rock Steady Boxing helps people maintain their physical independence, improve their quality of life, and restore confidence and dignity while we wait for a cure. Rock Steady Boxing empowers people with Parkinson's to "fight back" figuratively and literally.

Professional boxers condition for optimal agility, speed, muscular endurance, accuracy, hand-eye coordination, footwork, and overall strength to defend against and overcome opponents. At Rock Steady Boxing, Parkinson's is the opponent.

Researchers at institutions such as the University of Indianapolis and the Cleveland Clinic have validated physical and neurological improvement in Parkinson's patients participating in intense forced workouts. Studies have shown that those participating in the Rock Steady Boxing program can see a delay, reversal, and/or reduction in symptoms.

Getting the right kind of exercise is part of the battle, but equally important are the social and emotional benefits that people gain from Rock Steady:

- *We came to see we were more than "victims." We could help others and help ourselves!*
- *We didn't know how much we needed Rock Steady Boxing. Thanks to Rock Steady, both of us have a more positive outlook on our future.*
- *Today, I have a new lease on life. I am upbeat, happy, and optimistic—I have* hope. *I have taken control of this disease. It is not controlling me.*
- *My total well-being—morale, physical ability, and relationship with others—is better because of Rock Steady.*

Each month at the Indianapolis headquarters gym,

more than 230 people participate in boxing-inspired exercises. Exercises vary depending on the individual's fitness and progression of symptoms.

Today, there are hundreds of Rock Steady Boxing affiliate locations throughout the world.

Rock Steady Boxing is living its battle cry: "In this corner: Hope."

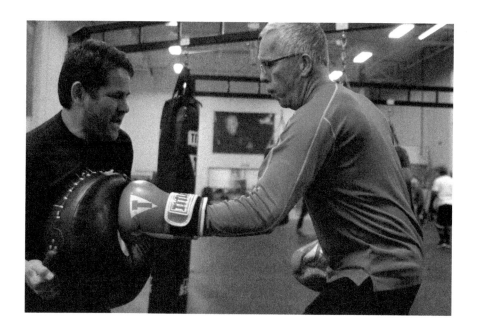

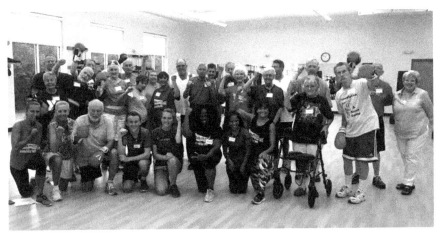

Rock Steady Boxing at the Hopkinsville YMCA, Kentucky

Start a Rock Steady Program
in Your Community

Since its inception, Rock Steady Boxing has enjoyed incredible media interest. Stories about Scott Newman, Parkinson's disease, and boxing as a way to improve the quality of life of a person with Parkinson's began to appear on national news outlets as early as 2008. Following each news story, Rock Steady Boxing received hundreds of phone calls from people all over the country who wanted to know where the Rock Steady Boxing affiliate in their community was. Until 2012, the answer was, "I'm sorry, but Rock Steady is only in Indianapolis."

In 2012, Rock Steady Boxing developed a Training Camp (the boxing term for seminar) to teach boxing coaches, personal trainers, therapists, people with Parkinson's, and people with an interest in helping people with Parkinson's the boxing skills, techniques, and specific ways that intense exercise affects Parkinson's. During this fun, interactive, and hands-on seminar, participants "guest coach" in classes and are inspired by the dedication of our boxers. Certification as a Rock Steady coach provides all the information needed to replicate the Rock Steady method in a hometown gym or facility.

In 2016, Rock Steady will launch an online certification program to again expand the opportunities for certification and for establishing community programs.

Rock Steady Boxing's mission is to educate as many people as possible about the benefits of intense exercise and the Rock Steady method, and to increase the number of safe and welcoming places for people with Parkinson's to exercise.

By the end of 2016, it is expected that there will be more than 300 affiliate locations throughout the world and that the Rock Steady method will be a worldwide movement in the fight against Parkinson's.

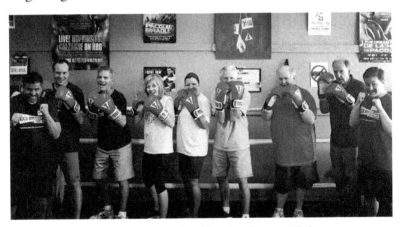

Rock Steady Boxing Birmingham, Alabama

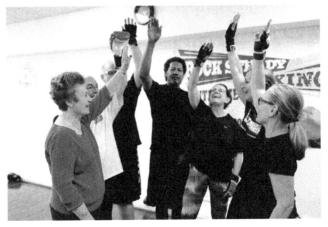

Rock Steady Boxing Central Jersey, New Jersey

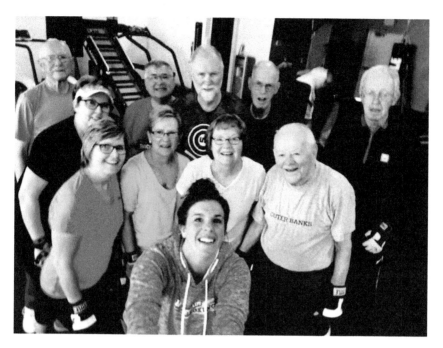

Rock Steady Boxing Columbia, Missouri

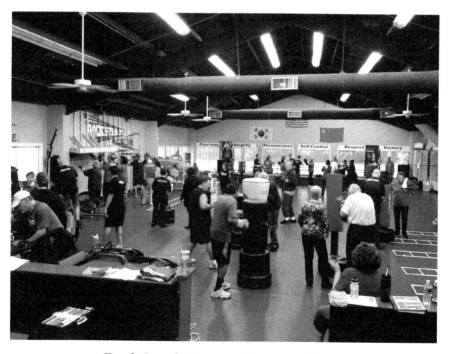

Rock Steady Boxing Houston, Texas

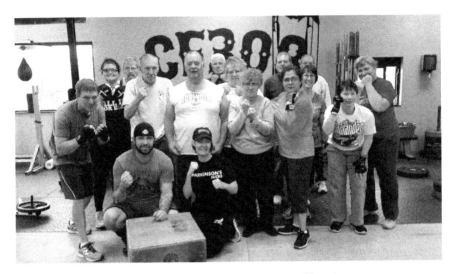

Rock Steady Boxing Peoria, Illinois

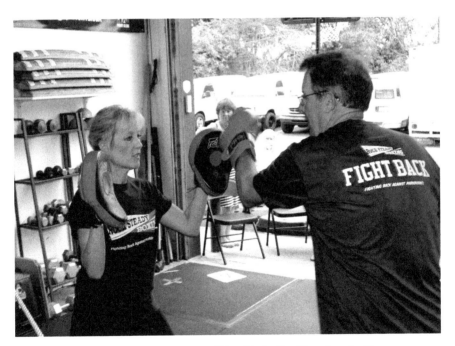

Rock Steady Boxing Rose City Rebels, Portland, Oregon

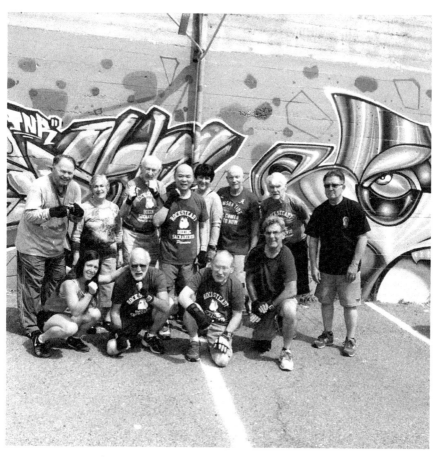

Rock Steady Boxing Sacramento, California

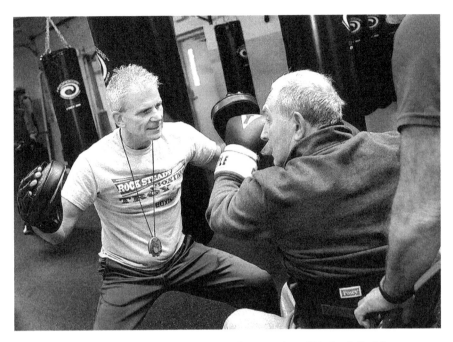

Rock Steady Boxing Troy at the Boxing Rink, Michigan

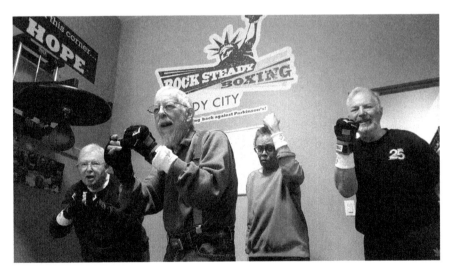

Rock Steady Boxing Windy City, Chicago, Illinois

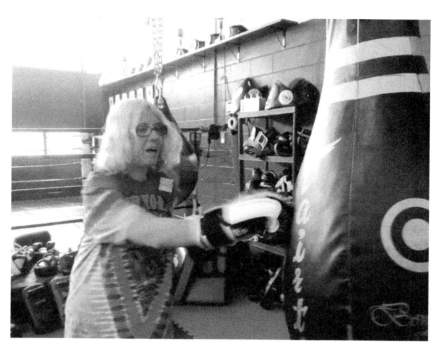

Rock Steady Boxing Toronto, Ontario, Canada

Support Rock Steady Boxing

Rock Steady Boxing is a nonprofit organization (EIN # 20-5113083) that depends upon the generosity of individual donors, local businesses, and corporations for support.

It's our mission to have a Rock Steady Boxing program in every community throughout the world so that when someone hears the words "You have Parkinson's disease," it will be followed with "and there's a gym down the street where you can fight back."

Your tax-deductible gifts will make this happen. You will have an impact on the lives of people with Parkinson's all over the world. It's your generosity that will grow and multiply this program.

You can donate online at www.rocksteadyboxing.org or send your check to **Rock Steady Boxing, 6847 Hillsdale Court, Indianapolis, IN 46250.**

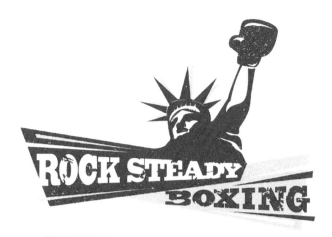

FIGHTING BACK AGAINST PARKINSON'S

The Rock Steady Logo

Rock Steady Boxing is often asked about the design of our logo—the Statue of Liberty embellished with a boxing glove. According to our founder, Scott Newman, the words inscribed on the Statue of Liberty, and the hope symbolized by her presence at Ellis Island, illustrate his dream that Rock Steady Boxing would be a beacon of light and hope for those suffering with Parkinson's disease.

Inscription on the Statue of Liberty
Give me your tired, your poor,
Your huddled masses yearning to breathe free,
The wretched refuse of your teeming shore.
Send these, the homeless, tempest-tost to me,
I lift my lamp beside the golden door!"
(*Author: Emma Lazarus*)

ABOUT THE WRITER

Julie Young is an award-winning freelance writer and author in the Indianapolis area who has written six books on local history, including *The Famous Faces of WTTV-4* and *Eastside Indianapolis: A Brief History*; two titles for the Complete Idiot's Guide series, including *The Complete Idiot's Guide to Catholicism*; and a young adult novel entitled *Fifteen Minutes of Fame*. Her work has been seen in a variety of local, regional, national, and international publications, including the *Indianapolis Star*, *Indianapolis Monthly*, *AAA Home & Away*, *Today's Catholic Teacher*, and CNN.com. She has appeared on *Hoosier History Live!* and *First Day* with Terri Stacy as well as the *Oprah Winfrey Show*. She lives with her family, and in her spare time, she coaches tennis for the National Junior Tennis League (NJTL).

About the Photographer

Marc Morrison (www.marcmorrison.com) is an Austin-based photographer who lives to visually create and collaborate with musicians, athletes, and everyday people. As a worldwide advertising photographer for more than 20 years, Marc has seen his commissions venture into various genres. He has photographed numerous advertising campaigns for major agencies Campbell Ewald; Purple Strategies, Inc., Design; Ogilvy & Mather; The Team; FleishmanHillard; and TMP Worldwide and for clients such as HBO, Chevrolet, Hess Corporation, BP, Petrofac, ExxonMobile, NIKE, and United Airlines.

His portraiture includes subjects from Merle Haggard and Lil Wayne to Fortune 500 CEOs and world leaders. Marc's work has appeared in countless outlets such as *Fortune, Forbes, The Verge, TIME, Rolling Stone, SPIN, New York Times, Golf Digest*, and *Sports Illustrated*.

Marc enjoys pushing boundaries yet understands how to achieve the client's vision. His ability to adapt to any situation, work within tight time frames, develop camaraderie with his subjects, and produce thought-provoking visuals sets him apart from other photographers. When he's not on the road, Marc is an avid mountain biker who loves to sail. He lives with his girlfriend and their three amazing rescue dogs.

Bibliography

Barbarosa, Dennis. "The Interview Issue: Scott Newman." *Indianapolis Business Journal.* 27 September 2014. http://www.ibj.com/articles/49695-the-interview-issue-scott-newman

Beck, David Alan. "Punching out Parkinson's at Rock Steady Boxing Gym." *Nuvo Weekly.* 14 February 2007. http://www.nuvo.net/indianapolis/punching-out-parkinsons-at-rock-steady-boxing-gym/Content?oid=1206980

Boracchi, Chiara. "La boxe per curare il Parkinson: nasce la prima palestra italiana." 16 March 2015. http://www.lifegate.it/persone/stile-di-vita/boxe-parkinson-prima-palestra-italiana

Canali, Roberto. "Un pugno al Parkinson." *Como Cronaca IL Giorno.* 20 March 2015. http://www.ilgiorno.it/como/longone-boxe-parkinson-1.774778

Cenci, Federico. "Un campione di pugilato in udienza dal Papa." *ZENIT.* 22 April 2015. https://it.zenit.org/articles/un-campione-di-pugilato-in-udienza-dal-papa/

Conley, Mikaela. "Rock Steady Gym Workouts Fight off Parkinson's Disease." *Northwest Parkinson's Foundation.* 23 February 2011. https://nwpf.org/stay-informed/news/2011/02/rock-steady-gym-workouts-fight-off-parkinsons-disease/

George, Chris. "Fighting Back." TBNWeekly.com. 24 November 2015. http://www.tbnweekly.com/editorial/health_news/content_articles/112415_hth-01.txt

Hetrick, Bruce. "Trials and Tribulations." *Indianapolis Monthly.* February 2003.

Le Verrier, Renne. "Yoga, Parkinson's and a Pair of Pink Gloves." PD Gladiators blog guest post. 6 January 2014.
http://pdgladiators.org/guest-post-yoga-parkinsons-and-a-pair-of-pink-gloves/

Latham, Aaron. "The Cowboy Chronicles." *New York.*
http://nymag.com/nymetro/arts/features/3840/

Mitchell, Kerry. "Fighting a Tough Foe." *Northwest Times of Indiana.* 6 August 2007.
http://www.nwitimes.com/niche/get-healthy/fighting-a-tough-foe/article_cb21fc7a-be6d-549c-8340-eef4310767c1.html

Newman, Scott. "My View: Battling Disease, Competition with a One-Two Punch." *Indianapolis Star.* 18 July 2007. http://eypadvisors.com/a-"can-do"-attitude/

Mayo Clinic. "Parkinson's disease."http://www.mayoclinic.org/diseases-conditions/parkinsons-disease/basics/definition/con-20028488

Pond, Steve. "A 'Perfect' Puzzle—Travolta's New Movie: How Much Is Real?" *Washington Post*. 6 June 1985. https://www.washingtonpost.com/archive/lifestyle/1985/06/06/a-perfect-puzzle-travoltas-new-movie-how-much-is-real/15aca350-5999-43b3-a261-2e72b6f33528/

"Region Native Kristy Follmar Helps Knock out Parkinson's Disease." *Northwest Times of Indiana*. 20 April 2008. https://nwpf.org/stay-informed/news/2008/04/region-native-kristy-follmar-helps-knock-out-parkinsons-disease/

Reporter, PA. "No Proof Muhammad Ali's Parkinson's Disease Caused by Boxing, Reveals Former Champion's Personal Doctor." *Daily Mail*. 2 November 2014. http://www.dailymail.co.uk/sport/boxing/article-2817592/No-proof-Muhammad-Ali-s-Parkinson-s-Disease-caused-boxing.html

Roda. "Boxe senza contatto per parkinsoniani, ecco I miei pogetti" *Sport Europa*. October 2015. https://issuu.com/sporteuropa/docs/sport_europa_-_ottobre_2015

Rubin, Susan M. "Parkinson's Disease in Women." American Parkinson Disease Association. http://www.apda-parkinson.org/parkinsons-disease-in-women/

Smilgis, Martha. "CBS Anchor Lesley Stahl and Writer Aaron Latham Have a Mixed-Media Marriage." *People*. 31 October 1977. Vol. 8. No. 8. http://www.people.com/people/archive/article/0,,20069431,00.html

Stahl, Lesley. "Fighting Back Against Parkinson's—in the Ring." *Sunday Morning*. CBS News. 8 November 2015 http://www.cbsnews.com/news/fighting-back-against-parkinsons-in-the-ring/3/

Ulrich, Nate. "In Wake of Tragedy, Follmar Returns to Boxing." *Northwest Times of Indiana*. 19 February 2009. http://www.nwitimes.com/sports/in-wake-of-tragedy-follmar-returns-to-boxing/article_6c7d8a07-86a0-57bb-afa0-d766b7c3be89.html

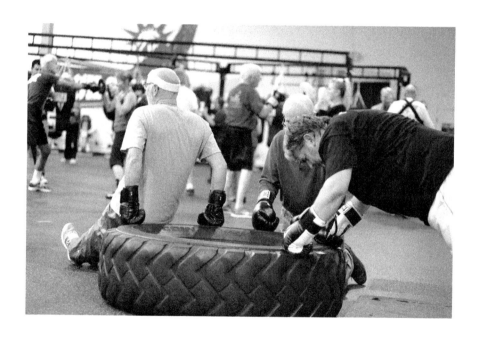

CPSIA information can be obtained
at www.ICGtesting.com
Printed in the USA
LVOW06s1345130617
537876LV00006B/9/P